THE PSYCHOLOGY OF SET

EKSPERIMENTAL'NYE OSNOVY PSIKHOLOGII USTANOVKI

ЭКСПЕРИМЕНТАЛЬНЫЕ ОСНОВЫ ПСИХОЛОГИИ УСТАНОВКИ

Other volumes in

INTERNATIONAL BEHAVIORAL SCIENCES SERIES

D. N. Uznadze
THE PSYCHOLOGY OF SET • *1966*

A. R. Luria
HIGHER CORTICAL FUNCTIONS IN MAN • *1966*

B. V. Zeigarnik
THE PATHOLOGY OF THINKING • *1965*

Albrecht Peiper
CEREBRAL FUNCTION IN INFANCY AND CHILDHOOD • *1964*

N. P. Bekhtereva
BIOPOTENTIALS OF CEREBRAL HEMISPHERES IN BRAIN TUMORS • *1962*

L. V. Krushinskii
ANIMAL BEHAVIOR: Its Normal and Abnormal Development • *1962*

G. Yu. Malis
Research on the ETIOLOGY OF SCHIZOPHRENIA • *1961*

M. S. Pevzner
OLIGOPHRENIA: Mental Deficiency in Children • *1961*

B. V. Andreev
SLEEP THERAPY IN THE NEUROSES • *1960*

In preparation:
S. M. Blinkov and I. I. Glezer
THE HUMAN BRAIN IN FIGURES AND TABLES
A Quantitative Handbook

THE INTERNATIONAL BEHAVIORAL SCIENCES SERIES

Editor: Joseph Wortis, M.D.

State University of New York, Downstate Medical Center, Brooklyn, New York

THE PSYCHOLOGY OF SET

Dmitrii Nikolaevich Uznadze

Georgian Institute of Psychology
Academy of Sciences of the Georgian SSR

Translated from the Russian by

Basil Haigh

Cambridge, England

SPRINGER SCIENCE+BUSINESS MEDIA, LLC
1966

This book is the product of many years of experimental research by the late Soviet psychologist D. N. Uznadze (1886-1950) and the group of Georgian psychologists whom he directed.

ISBN 978-1-4899-4763-5 ISBN 978-1-4899-4761-1 (eBook)
DOI 10.1007/978-1-4899-4761-1

The original Russian text was published by the Academy of Sciences of the Georgian SSR for the D. N. Uznadze Institute of Psychology in Tiflis in 1961.

ЭКСПЕРИМЕНТАЛЬНЫЕ ОСНОВЫ
ПСИХОЛОГИИ УСТАНОВКИ

Дмитрий Николаевич Узнадзе

Library of Congress Catalog Card Number 65-21186

Originally published by Consultants Bureau in 1966
Softcover reprint of the hardcover ist edition 1966

Foreword

This volume is a translation of a Russian book entitled "Eksperimental'nye osnovy psikhologii ustanovki," literally "experimental basis of the psychology of set." In fact, the Russian book — and therefore the translation — comprises two monographs by the late Dmitrii Nikolaevich Uznadze; the first carries the above-mentioned title and the second is "Osnovnye polozheniya teorii ustanovkii," or literally "basic principles of the theory of set." The first of these monographs was originally published in Georgian in 1949, although the book was originally written in Russian. The printing in 1961 of the Russian volume on which this translation is based was the first publication in Russian of the original monograph and the first publication in any form of the second monograph. The Russian 1961 edition was prepared by an editorial board under the chairmanship of A. S. Prangishvili, a close coworker of Uznadze, who is responsible for the "Notes from the Editor" on page 249 of this volume.

New York
April 1966

Joseph Wortis

Preface

The basic idea behind the present book—the concept of relative set—was one which I first formulated twenty-five years ago ("Impersonalia," Chveni Metsniereba, No. 1, 1923). From that time until the present, this idea has been continuously and logically developed. Progress became particularly rapid after my pupils and colleagues began to take part in its development. In 1933 and 1943, two collections ("Data Concerning the Psychology of Set") were published, in which investigations carried out in the Psychological Laboratory of the University were described.

The literature on the many aspects of set is now fairly extensive, and this affords me the opportunity of presenting to the reader the fundamental principles of the theory in the form in which it appears to me in the present stage of investigation. I must point out that the present book bears the imprint of all my colleagues insofar as the subject is concerned with the problematics of set. I take this opportunity of thanking all of them, especially N. Eliava and A. Prangishvili, who were of great assistance in preparing the final text.

D. N. Uznadze

Introduction

The whole complex of theories describing the processes of mental activity is based upon the grouping of its manifestations into three categories—sensation, cognition, and volition—which are the fundamental units of traditional classification. In the history of psychology, of course, there has been more than one attempt made to explain mental phenomena in terms of different basic categories, but the traditional classification remains dominant.

The natural question is: What is it that makes these three categories fundamental? Evidently, it is simply that without exception they are conscious processes—cognition, like sensation or volition, is equally a phenomenon of consciousness. The individual who performs any act of cognition or volition or who experiences any emotion shows by certain accompanying actions that these are fully conscious mental phenomena. According to this point of view, it is perfectly clear that mind and consciousness are precisely the same thing: Everything mental is conscious, and everything conscious must necessarily be mental.

Since this is the traditional and most widespread conception of the nature of the mind, we may then ask how this theory deals with the problem of mental development.

Obviously, there is no room within its framework to accommodate the concept of development. Since mental activity can take place only in the presence of conscious processes, we must assume that the mind is completely divorced from everything devoid of consciousness, from everything material, and constitutes an absolutely original sphere of reality, which rules out any possibility that mind and matter may have an influence upon each other. Because traditional theory provides no grounds for assuming interaction of mental and physical, the problem of what their relationship is can be solved only in terms of the concept of so-called psychophysical parallelism, which is a perfectly natural and logical conclusion according to the above assumptions.

However, if parallelism is accepted as a legitimate concept, we are forced to conclude that thought is impotent before the problems which it brings to light. Therefore, the idea of parallelism cannot be accepted as correct. It must be replaced by something more acceptable, and we cannot assume that mind and consciousness are identical. Instead, we must assume the existence of the mind in some manifestation not coincident with consciousness, and it must be added, not antecedent to it.

Within the literature of psychology can be found another trend of thought addressed to the solution of the problem here engaging us—the relationship between mind and consciousness—in a completely different manner. This is the assumption that mental life does not consist entirely of conscious mental experiences, but rather that it encompasses a wide field of reality, of which the zone of consciousness is only an insignificant part—in brief, that mind and consciousness are not the same at all and need not overlap. On the contrary, there is reason to suppose the existence of a second and in any event no less important area of mental life known as the "unconscious" or "subconscious" mind, which occupies a considerable part of the field of mental activity. From this point of view, certain phenomena may be regarded as mental but not necessarily conscious. The mind includes two large, equally essential components—conscious experience and unconscious experience. This is the basic viewpoint of the so-called psychology of the unconscious.

According to this concept, it might be assumed that the mind passes through two stages of development in the course of its functioning: first the unconscious stage and then the conscious. However, the psychology of the unconscious is far removed from this idea, because its adherents in no way consider that the terms "conscious" and "unconscious" merely represent two successive stages in the ontogenesis of a single mind. Certainly, I have known instances of an unconscious state becoming a conscious state, wherein the conscious arises out of the unconscious, but this is not the one essential path which mental processes must follow in order to reach the conscious state. The sequence of events is frequently seen to occur in the opposite order; that is, a conscious state becomes unconscious. Consequently, it must be emphasized that the unconscious is not necessarily a stage of development which is followed by the stage of consciousness.

What this in fact means with respect to the psychology of the unconscious is made clear by an analysis of the unconscious mental process itself: What does the term "unconscious" really mean? How shall we describe it; how shall we define the quality of this state? Let us assume that a subject develops some desire that he regards as unsuitable, or perhaps even shameful, for some reason or other. What happens in such a case? The psychology of the unconscious here falls back upon the concept of repression, and it is assumed that the subject "represses" the desire from his consciousness, not eradicating it once and for all, but merely relegating it to the depths of his unconscious. In this repressed, and now unconscious, state, the desire is not consciously perceived or experienced by the subject, but it is not forever disposed of. The subject still retains his desire to some degree and it continues to act upon him, but in such a way that he knows nothing about it. And so, according to the theory, this is how one very considerable part of the unconscious mind is created.

But what happens to this mental process in the unconscious state? Is it modified to some degree, or is the transition from the conscious state into the unconscious a simple mechanical displacement of the process not affecting its real nature at all? How are these questions answered according to the psychology of the unconscious?

First of all, we must recall what happens when mental processes move in the opposite direction, that is, during the change from the unconscious state into the conscious.

It is obvious that before a particular state can become conscious it must manifest itself in the form of one of the familiar conscious states, let us say as some emotional state, a feeling of fear, for example.

In accordance with this concept, there is no doubt that the unconscious experience, both at the moment of its appearance and after it has become conscious, remains essentially the same: A conscious state may become unconscious, and, conversely, an unconscious state may return to the consciousness. This of course does not mean that these transitions must necessarily take place; the important issue is the presence or absence of the attribute of consciousness in a given case.

In the psychology of the unconscious, the unconscious mental state is defined only negatively, that is, as a mental state lacking consciousness. The theory cannot supply a positive definition, and so the process is regarded as being that which upon acquiring the sign of consciousness becomes an ordinary phenomenon of consciousness. The unconscious consists of those processes outside consciousness and without consciousness. Positive definition is thought to be impossible.

It is obvious that this concept of the unconscious is of no value in solving the problem with which we are concerned—that of mental development. The unconscious as described in terms of the psychology of the unconscious is never a stage in the development of the mind, preceding and preparing for the appearance of conscious mental experience. The unconscious and the conscious are identical, and therefore they both represent the same level of development.

In a word, since it is obvious that the psychology of the unconscious is of no use in interpreting the unconscious state as a stage of mental development, it is also obvious that the concept of mental development is itself completely foreign to this type of psychology, in which mental activity is regarded as a purely subjective process, conscious or unconscious.

Of course, there have been many attempts made to establish the fact of mental development in both ontogenesis and phylogenesis; however, such investigations have always been concerned with the development of mental activity as a conscious process. So far, the question of what stages precede the appearance of the conscious mind has largely been ignored in bourgeois science. The real point is that the question has never arisen in traditional psychology, since from the first it has been dogmatically postulated that the conscious mind is just as primary, original, and basic as physical, material existence. The mind which participates in acts of cognition, sensation, and volition is assumed to be a primary datum; its reduction to earlier levels of development is inconceivable. At any rate, the prehistory of the mind as such has never been the object of serious scientific research in traditional psychology.

However, if it is assumed that the mind does develop in several stages, and that it is not a predetermined entity, then there is no reason to believe that it exists only in the form of conscious manifestations. On the contrary, it must rather be assumed that there is a form of mental activity which necessarily precedes consciousness; in other words, there is a preconscious stage of mental development.

V.I. Lenin pointed out that this hypothesis rests on firm foundations. In his work "Materialism and Empiricocriticism," he states that "as a clearly expressed form, perception is associated only with the higher forms of matter (organic matter)" and also that "at the foundations of the edifice of matter we can only postulate the existence of a faculty similar to that of preception."*

So far as I can judge, Lenin did not elaborate upon this idea in his later works, or at least he had no reason to use it in connection with psychology. However, the idea is of considerable philosophical import, and it is one of the more urgent tasks of Marxist psychology that this thesis be employed in concrete psychological investigation. The essential problem to be faced is how the mind really develops, and consequently what are the stages preceding consciousness.†

What, precisely, is the preconscious stage of mental development? This question, of fundamental importance in psychology, can only be answered on the basis of experimental investigation. Because this problem has not been given its due attention, there is no direct answer to be found among the achievements of psychology. Essentially, the question is here being raised for the first time, and later we shall try to answer it. We shall find that the stage of development preceding consciousness in that of set fixing, which we will now proceed to study.

*V. I. Lenin, "Materialism and Empiricocriticism," Partizdat TsK VKP (b), 1936, p. 30.
†See editor's note.

Contents

Introduction to the Theory of Set

I. ENUNCIATION OF THE PROBLEM

1. The Illusion of Volume

Let us take two objects of different weights, but absolutely identical in all other respects, e.g., two balls, one of which is obviously heavier than the other, but equal in volume and all other properties. If we give these balls to a subject and ask him to compare their volumes, as a rule he will answer that the heavier ball is smaller than the lighter. Generally, the greater the difference in weight, the more common is the illusion of disparate volume. It may be assumed that the illusion arises from the fact that as an object increases in weight it usually also increases in volume; the heavier ball should be larger than the lighter ball. In the absence of such an actual increase in volume, the subject perceives the heavier ball to be even smaller than it really is.

In the process of experimentation, however, it is better to use objects different in volume rather than weight, that is, to present repeatedly to a subject two objects of different volumes so that one, say, the smaller, is always placed in his right hand and the other, the larger, in his left hand. After a certain number of repetitions, usually 10 to 15, the subject is given two balls of equal volume and asked to compare them. Usually, he will not say that they are equal; rather, it seems to him that one is clearly larger than the other. In the overwhelming majority of cases, the illusion will be one of contrast; the ball that seems the larger to him is the one he holds in the hand which held the smaller ball in the previous presentations. This phenomenon occurs much more distinctly and more often when volume rather than weight is the critical factor. The illusion of disparate volume may also be centered upon the hand which held the larger ball in the preliminary presentations; that is, the subject, upon being given identical balls, may continue to have the impression that he has a larger ball in the same hand as before. In this case, we refer to the illusion as the "phenomenon of assimilation."

However, volume is not only perceived haptically, as in the experiments above, but also visually, and therefore we are interested in how the illusion of volume may arise when both factors are considered.

In this series of experiments, we tachystoscopically presented the subject with two circles, one obviously larger than the other, and asked him to compare them and say which was larger. After a sufficient number of similar presentations, we turned to the critical experiment, tachystoscopically showing him two identical circles to compare in size.

The results were as follows: The circles were perceived illusorily, nearly always as illusions of contrast; direct assimilation was rarely observed. We shall not describe the experimental results further, except to mention that sometimes there was nearly a 100% illusion rate [68].

2. The Illusion of the Strength of Pressure

Besides the illusion of volume, we have also found several other related phenomena, particularly an illusion of pressure (1929).

Here, the subject is given two successive stimuli by means of a baresthesiometer—first a strong one and then a comparatively weak one. This is repeated 10 to 15 times. The experiments are designed to create in the subject a deep impression of this particular sequence of stimulation in preparation for the critical experiment to follow, in which he is given two stimuli of equal pressure to compare.

The usual result of the experiments was that the subject felt the critical stimuli as different rather than equal; the first pressure stimulus seemed to be greater than the second. As shown in Table I, illusions were much more common than correct perceptions.

As in the previous series of experiments, we were dealing with both symmetric and asymmetric illusions, the latter being more frequently observed, as before—that is, the equal experimental stimuli were perceived as unequal; stimulation on the side receiving greater pressure in the preliminary experiments seemed relatively weaker in the critical experiment (illusion of contrast). Under some conditions, however, the subject judged the critical stimulus to the

TABLE I

Reaction	+	–	=	?
Illusion of pressure, in %	45.6	25.0	15.0	14.4

+ Number of cases of contrast
– Number of assimilations
= Number of correct impressions
? Number of uncertain responses
These signs have the same meaning in all the subsequent tables.

side preliminarily given the stronger stimulus as continuing to be of greater pressure (assimilation).

We found that 70.6% of the perceptions in the critical experiments were illusions. Consequently, it is quite clear that phenomena analogous to the illusion of volume also occur in the perception of pressure, which differs significantly from perception of volume in the structure of its receptor.

3. The Illusion of Hearing

Our next experiments dealt with auditory impressions. In preliminary experiments, subjects received pairs of auditory impressions by means of the "falling apparatus" (Fallapparat), with the first member of each pair being much stronger than the second. After 10 to 15 repetitions, the critical experiments were performed by presentation of equal stimuli which the subjects were asked to compare.

The results are shown in Table II, where it may be seen that illusions reached 76% of the total of critical perceptions. Here, as in the experiments on the illusion of pressure (Table I), there were more assimilative illusions than usual, especially in comparison to those instances where illusions of contrast frequently rose to 100% of the total. It must be assumed that in both series of experiments a relevant factor in the increase of assimilations was the consecutive presentation of stimuli; that is, the subject was

TABLE II

	+	–	=	?
Auditory assimilation in %	57.0	19.0	21.0	3.0

to compare stimuli received one after the other rather than simultaneously. We shall try below to explain why this is so.

The results obtained in these experiments show conclusively that phenomena analogous to illusions of volume also occur in auditory perception.

4. The Illusion of Illumination

As early as 1930, I suggested [66] that the initial overassessment of the degree of illumination or darkening observed during adaptation to darkness might belong to the same category of phenomena as the perceptual illusions described above. This suggestion was subsequently confirmed in my laboratory by the following experiments:

The subject was asked to compare the degree of illumination of two circles, one of which was much brighter than the other. In preliminary presentations (10 to 15), the dark circle was always shown first; in the critical experiment, the subject was presented with two equally bright circles and asked to compare them. The results of these experiments (see Table III) show conclusively that, because of the influence of preliminary presentations, the critical circles are not perceived as equally bright; the illusion rate was greater than 73%.

5. The Illusion of Number

Given suitable conditions, similar phenomena occur in the comparison of quantitative relationships:

Preliminary exposures (10 to 15) consist of showing the subject two circles, one of which contains many dots and the other few; in the critical experiment, both circles contain the same number of dots, but the subject generally sees many more in the circle previously containing fewer dots.

6. The Illusion of Weight

Fechner (1860) and Müller and Schumann (1889) observed a phenomenon similar to those we have described which later became known as the illusion of weight. It occurs as follows:

If a subject is instructed to lift a pair of objects obviously differing in weight several times in succession, with the heavier being always in the right hand, he will manifest a resultant state of perceiving equal objects as unequal; the object in the hand

TABLE III

Reaction	+	–	=	?
Illusion of illumination	56.6	16.6	21.6	5.2

previously holding the lighter object will seem heavier than that in the other hand. Therefore, illusions essentially similar to those occuring in our experiments also arise in the perception of weight.

7. Attempts to Explain These Phenomena

A. Müller's Theory

If we examine the results of these experiments, it becomes apparent that in all of them we are dealing with essentially the same phenomenon: All the illusions described are of the same character, and they arise in completely analogous conditions; consequently, they must be variants of the same phenomenon. However, since Müller's theory deals specifically with illusions in the perception of weight, it is too limited in scope to account for the illusions arising in other sensory modalities.

Müller's argument is as follows: When we give a subject a pair of objects of different weight to lift, he eventually becomes habituated to exerting a stronger muscular impulse to lift the first (heavier) object than the second. Because his right hand is accustomed to lifting a heavier object after 10 to 15 repetitions, he will continue to exert a greater lifting force on this side even when we give him two objects of equal weight. Therefore, the object in his right hand will be lifted faster and more easily than that in his left, seeming to "fly up into the air."

According to this theory, the psychological basis of the illusion is the sensation of comparative rapidity in lifting the weight; if it apparently "jumps up into the air" it seems light, but if it comes up more slowly and seems "glued to the table" the sensation is of a heavier object. Were it not for these impressions, the subject would not experience the illusion of weight.

However, since analogous phenomena occur in instances where there could not possibly be any impressions of "jumping up" or "being glued down" (illusions of volume, pressure, sound, illumination, number, having little or no connection with any specific peripheral processes), it is obvious that a theory based on the specific features of weight perception is not acceptable as an explanation of the entire category of illusions. The illusion of pressure arises from tactile sensations, the illusion of volume from haptic and visual sensations, and that of weight from muscular sensations, but they are all manifestations of one phenomenon of perception. Therefore, we must reject Müller's theory and look elsewhere for an answer.

The first question to arise is whether we can find some common basis for the activity of the individual sensory modalities in the conditions of our experiments.

B. The Theory of "Disappointed Expectation"

In the literature of psychology a theory is described which apparently answers our question completely—the theory of "disappointed expectation." Admittedly, the analogies to the illusion of weight, as we have described them, were not yet known when this theory was formulated, since they were first published much later in a study of the basis of this particular illusion [66]. However, the theory merits all the more attention now because the presence of such analogies indicates the need for a formal, unified explanation.

The theory of "disappointed expectation" explains the illusion of weight as follows: As a result of repeatedly lifting the weight (or, to apply to our experiments, of the repeated action of visual, auditory, or other forms of impressions), the subject develops the expectation that the object in one particular hand will always be heavier. Because this expectation is disappointed in the critical experiment, he underestimates the weight of the object and considers it lighter than the object in his other hand. This is how the illusion of contrast arises in this instance; in appropriate circumstances, the other analogues of this phenomenon which we have discovered will also arise in the same way.

The basic advantage of this theory over Müller's theory is that it accounts for the possibility that our phenomena may occur in any condition where there may be "disappointed expectation," which agrees with our findings that the illusion is not restricted to any one sensory modality but rather has a much wider distribution.

Nevertheless, this theory cannot be accepted. In the first place, it does not explain why in some cases the illusion is one of contrast while in others it is one of assimilation. Next, there is no reason to think that the subject in fact "expects" that he will continue to receive stimuli in the pattern of the preliminary experiments;

the impossibility of such an "expectation" is shown by the persistence of the illusion after one or two exposures to stimuli quite different from those which he might be assumed to "expect." In our experiments, illusions continued to appear not only after one or two trials, but even in subsequent exposures.

Even without these objections, we cannot reach a final decision about the theory of "disappointed expectation" without first attempting to verify it, experimentally, if possible.

We have carried out experiments specifically designed to test the theory, employing the hypnotic trance as a suitable condition for investigation of the problem because it indicates the existence of a state of rapport between the subject and the experimenter.

Preliminary experiments were performed while the subjects were in the hypnotic state. We put ordinary balls, one large and one small, into their hands and, on the basis of our rapport with them, directed that they compare the size of the balls. Although we knew that the usual posthypnotic amnesia would occur, we made a special point of suggesting to the subjects that they deliberately forget everything that happened while they were hypnotized. Each subject was then taken into another room and wakened; a short time later, when fully awake, he was subjected to the critical experiment, in which he was given two balls of equal size to compare.

Almost every subject thought that the ball in his left hand (the hand in which the larger ball had been placed earlier) was appreciably smaller than that in his right. This proves that the illusion may also occur when there is no possibility that the subject could have any "expectations" resulting from the influence of the preliminary experiments, since he had no idea of what had taken place during hypnosis. Therefore, the theory of "disappointed expectation" does not explain our observations.

8. Set as the Basis of These Illusions

What, then, does determine the behavior described in these experiments? Clearly, the decisive factor is that common to all experimental conditions, whether the specific object of our concern be the illusion arising from haptic or visual sensations in volume perception or the illusions in the perception of relative weight, pressure, illumination, or number. The aspects which distinguish one experiment from another are not the important ones.

Of course, all these diverse tests must have a common basis if there is to be a single explanation to account for the results.

And, in fact, each of them was concerned with the definition of quantitative relationships—in one instance with the relationship in size of two balls and in others with the relative intensity of pressure or weight or with relative numbers of objects. Solution of the problems always required quantitative comparison.

However, these relationships did not represent abstract categories in our experiments. In each instance, the subject was to determine the specific relationship between two objects; for example, in the problem of the size of the circles, he was first given two unequal circles several times and then two equal circles in the critical exposure. In other tests, he was given quite different experimental stimuli—two unequal impressions of pressure or number followed by the respective equal critical stimuli. Despite the diversity of experimental material, he was always faced with the problem of finding a quantitative relationship. However, he never experienced it in any generalized form. Even though the quantitative relationship was the one general characteristic of the various experiments, the subject did not perceive it abstractly but rather always gave it concrete expression.

How does this take place? We must assume that our preliminary presentations are of decisive importance in this process. During the repeated presentation of objects, the subject acquires some form of internal state which prepares him for the perception of subsequent presentations. There can be no doubt that this internal state does in fact exist and that it actually does arise from the effect of repeated preliminary presentations: It is only necessary to make the critical presentation without preliminary preparation to see that he perceives the relationship correctly. Therefore, the reason why identical objects seem unequal in the usual course of experimentation is that this is the manner in which objects were perceived in the preliminary presentations.

How can this be explained? We have seen that there are no grounds for suggesting that the subject has any "expectation" concerning the relationship of stimuli to come or even that he "expects" to receive stimuli recognizable as being the same kind experienced in preliminary presentations.

However, we know that any attempt to explain this state of affairs on the basis of as yet unproved psychological factors will be unsuccessful. We must therefore direct our attention to special experiments in order to solve the problem. These are our previously described experiments with hypnosis, the results of which are given in Table IV.

TABLE IV

Reaction	+	−	=
16 subjects	82%	17%	1%

Obviously, these results are basically the same as those obtained in ordinary experimental conditions (Table I): Despite the posthypnotic amnesia which left the subject completely unaware of his having been given repeated preliminary sensations of holding a large ball in one hand and a small ball in the other, he nevertheless perceived equal balls as unequal in the critical experiment. The illusion of volume appeared in this instance, also.

What do these results tell us? They demonstrate conclusively that it makes no difference whether the subject knows anything about the preliminary experiments or not; in either case he is under the influence of a state which completely determines the outcome of the critical experiment. Although this state can in no degree be called conscious, it is definitely a fully active, and therefore quite real, factor in directing and determining the quality of consciousness. The subject may know nothing of his previous experiences, but their effect on the critical experiment is manifested in no uncertain manner.

Can it be doubted after this that there exists and acts in the mind of our subject a factor which could not conceivably be present in consciousness—that a state which therefore may be described as extraconscious has, in these circumstances, a decisive effect on the nature and course of conscious mental activity?

But does this mean that we have to accept the existence of the "unconscious" mind and so, by extension of its limits, find therein a place for the mental process observed in our experiments? Certainly not! In the special discussion of the problem of the unconscious which follows, we shall show that the widely prevalent theories of the unconscious usually make no distinction in principle between conscious and unconscious mental processes. They are thought to differ only with respect to whether the attribute of consciousness is present or absent; both have essentially the same nature. An unconscious phenomenon made conscious is no different than any other ordinary manifestation of consciousness. We, however, are not concerned with differences of this sort, nor with those specific processes which are outside the limits of consciousness only in the sense that they happen to lack its attributes.

The problem here is concerned with two different aspects of the mind, each representing a specific and independent level of mental development endowed with its own specific characteristics. The results of our experiments have made the early, preconscious stage of mental development accessible to scientific analysis.

The state which develops in our subjects as a result of preliminary experiments clearly cannot be described as any of the phenomena of consciousness. However, since the distinguishing feature of this state is that it prepares for or at least precedes the appearance of certain conscious manifestations, we might say that we can discern in it a peculiar tendency toward some of the intrinsic features of consciousness. The most descriptive name for this state is set, for the following reasons: First, it exists in the subject as an integral state. It is not a quality of consciousness, not an isolated mental quality to be contrasted with other conscious qualities or related to them in this sense. Second, rather than simply being one of the various characteristics of mental activity, it is a determining factor in the dynamics of the mind. Finally, it is not manifested as a definite aspect of consciousness but as an integral trend directed toward a definite activity. In a word, the set is more exactly a complete entity than it is any individual experience—it is the initial, fundamental reaction to a situation where there is a problem to be considered and solved.

According to this definition, all the illusions previously described are manifestations of the activity of the set. The state which arises in the subject as a result of the influence of objective stimuli (for example, the balls of different sizes used in our investigations) is not one of the processes of consciousness and cannot therefore be formulated as a limited mental function; instead, it is best described as the subject's set in a particular direction because of its distinctive influence upon him.

Being an integral state, this set lies at the basis of the absolutely determinate mental phenomena arising in consciousness. It does not in any way follow these phenomena, but, on the contrary, it may be said to prepare for their appearance, to determine their course and composition.

In order to study the set, it is desirable that we be able to observe its functioning for a reasonably long time. Therefore, it is important to fix it to the required degree, which is the purpose of our repeated presentation of experimental stimuli to the subject. We usually designate these repeated experiments as fixing or setting experiments and the set arising from their influence as a fixed set.

The following experiments were carried out to confirm our hypotheses:

As usual, we gave the subject two balls of different size in the preliminary series, or setting series, as we shall call it in the future. The only new factor introduced was in the critical experiments. Before, the critical objects had been two balls equal in size to the smaller of the setting objects. Here, however, they were larger than the larger of the setting objects. In another series of experiments, the critical objects were cubes, and in a series of optical experiments several different shapes were used.

The results agreed with our predictions. The critical objects appeared unequal to the subjects, and so the illusion occurs in these circumstances, also.

In the case where the critical objects were balls larger than either of the setting objects, a new value was introduced. And in the experiments with pairs of different shapes, the set formed in response to a different kind of material influenced the critical perception. This proves that the material used in the setting experiments is not an essential factor and that the set is produced purely on the basis of their relationship, which remains constant regardless of the variation in material and whatever sensory modalities are involved.

Still more striking results are obtained along the samc lines if the setting experiments themselves, rather than the critical experiments, are performed with pairs of different figures varying substantially from each other in size [99].

The subject is tachystoscopically given a series of figures, first one large and one small triangle and then squares, hexagons, and various other figures in pairs and in the same order. Briefly, the fixing experiments are so designed that the subject receives only a certain relationship repeatedly—a large figure on the right and a small figure on the left, or vice versa. The figures are changed with each presentation.

When the experiments are carried out with only the large-small relationship constant, the subjects develop a set to this relationship and nothing else. In the critical experiments, they are given a pair of identical figures (for example, circles, ellipses, or squares) to compare.

What are the results of these experiments? We shall discuss only those of immediate interest to our problem. We find that, despite the continuous change in the setting figures, while maintaining the same relationship between them, there is no doubt that the usual illusion of the set does develop. In some cases, the subjects do not notice that the critical figures are identical; moreover, the dominant form of illusion in this instance also is the phenomenon of contrast.

It should be pointed out, however, that in abstraction from concrete material, that is, in the experiments which we are describing, the action of the set is generally less effective than when the fixing and critical figures are very similar or identical. But this does not mean that the relationship between the figures does not have to be assessed when they are identical in the critical and fixing experiments. The problem in such a case remains essentially the same. However, it is quite obvious that these experiments are less effective in the case of complete abstraction from the qualitative attributes of the related objects.

By way of conclusion we can say that the phenomena we have discovered point unequivocably to the presence of not only conscious processes but also preconscious processes in our mental activity; and, as we shall show, these may be described as the field of the set.

9. Perception by Contrast

There remains a problem to be solved before we can finally assume that it is in fact the set which is involved in these experiments.

The term "set" implies a definite state of preparation to solve a problem in which the manner of solution is predetermined. In our experiments, the set is modelled in the process of the preliminary presentations in the direction that, for example, the balls on the left must be larger than those on the right; however, the subsequent critical presentation of the experimental object frequently shows that this hypothesis is incorrect. On the contrary, a completely opposite result is obtained: The ball on the left appears much smaller, not larger, than that on the right. The presence of illusions of contrast, so often observed in our experiments, casts doubt on our hypothesis that it is in fact the set and not something else which is investigated.

What explanation can be given of the development of illusions in contrast to the set suggested in our experiments? In the first place, it is evident that in these experiments we must be dealing with the activity of the set, because, as mentioned above, the sole cause for the appearance of illusions is the effect of experiments with unequal objects prior to the presentation of identical critical objects. Without these preceding presentations, there is usually no illusion. Consequently, these presentations are necessarily an essential condition for the appearance of illusion, and all that we can assume is that a state of preparedness for the perception of all these objects as unequal is produced in the subject under the influence of the repeated fixing experiments. There would have been no doubt that this preparedness could be interpreted as the set if we had observed, not a phenomenon of contrast, but a phenomenon of assimilation, in harmony with it.

Special experiments which we carried out to verify this possibility of illusions of assimilation were as follows: The subjects received as fixing objects circles which, as the series progressed, became increasingly different from each other in area. We started by presenting circles 25 and 26 mm in diameter, followed these with 24 and 26 mm circles, and finally presented 22 and 26 mm circles. The results of these experiments are given in Table V.

These results show that the reactions given by our subjects to presentation of the stimuli were partly assimilative and partly contrasting (not counting instances when the stimuli were interpreted as equal). The distribution of these reactions is interesting. We can see this distribution better the greater the quantitative difference between the fixing objects, and — which is particularly interesting — the greater the difference between these circles, the higher the incidence of contrast, and, conversely, the smaller the difference between these circles, the higher the incidence of assimilation. Particular stress must be laid on the fact that in our

TABLE V

Stimulus	–	+	=
25–26 mm	68%	28%	4%
24–26 mm	33.7%	50%	16.3%
22–26 mm	25.1%	58%	16.6%

experiments a specific size relationship between the setting figures was found which proved most advantageous for the demonstration of assimilation. This occurred with the 25 and 26 mm circles. With this relationship, assimilations amounted to 68% of all cases. It must be remembered that, in general, the smaller the difference in size between the setting figures, the greater the number of assimilative perceptions. This observation is interesting in this particular instance because it shows conclusively that in our experiments we were in fact dealing with the set, which may act directly only by an assimilative mechanism.

On the other hand, we are not dealing only with assimilations in these experiments. On the contrary, the number of contrasting perceptions is by no means insignificant. Moreover, in the overwhelming majority of cases, namely, when the difference in size of the setting objects is comparatively great, these phenomena begin to assume not just a predominant place, but an exclusive place: In these conditions, assimilation is hardly ever seen. Therefore, we must explain as far as possible why in the presence of a set having a definite direction we obtain so many reactions opposite to this set. Assuming that perception by contrast arises most often when the difference between the setting objects is obviously great, we must conclude that in these conditions a factor interfering with the realization of the existing set must begin to operate. When two distinctly different objects are repeatedly presented, this evidently produces in the subject an appropriate set — a state of preparedness to receive in his hands distinctly different objects. However, he actually receives objects of the same size. This situation, it must be assumed, is so different from that to which he has developed a set that he is unable to perceive it on the basis of this set. There can be only one natural result of this: The subject must eradicate the obviously unsuitable set and try to perceive the new impression correctly. If, however, we assume that in general there can be no perception without the presence of corresponding sets, it becomes clear that instead of eradicating an inadequate set the subject must develop a new set more in line with the situation. We find that this becomes possible only after a certain time. Until then, the new set arising in place of the existing and so obviously unsuitable set is opposite to it, so that the subject perceives the situation on the basis of this objectively unfounded, but also unfixed, opposite set. However, it dies away comparatively quickly, and a new set gradually becomes established which enables the subject to perceive correctly the stimuli presented to him. And so the subject gradually becomes adapted to the impressions acting upon him [66].

These hypotheses concerning the origin of contrasting perceptions may appear somewhat artificial. However, there are additional arguments supporting them, and we shall discuss them next.

The problematical aspect in this particular instance is the fact of contrasting perception itself. What is the real source of contrast, when the influence of the set must essentially be entirely assimilative? The most important feature of these experiments is that we are dealing with quantitative relationships: The problem is always to compare phenomena in relation to the strength of pressure, weight, volume, and so on – that is, with respect to factors which can be expressed in quantitative units. We know, however, that contrast is a property confined to quantitatively related phenomena, and this category is usually not applied to any other sphere of reality. If, therefore, we try to investigate the set in terms of qualitative rather than quantitative relationships, then perhaps we shall find a completely different picture.

In the subsequent account we shall many times have occasion to discuss the set in relation to the world of qualitatively different phenomena. At this point, I shall mention one of the experimental methods used in studying this category.

If a subject is asked to read, let us say, a text written in Latin letters, and soon afterward is shown a series of disconnected Russian words composed of letters common to both Cyrillic and Latin scripts (for example, B O P), for a time he will read these Russian sounds as if they were printed in Latin letters.

There is no doubt that an appropriate set is activated in the subject when he reads the Latin words, and when he is given a Russian word, that is, a word in a familiar language, he reads it as if it were a Latin word. Only after a certain period of time does the subject begin to realize his mistake.

These experiments clearly show that in the course of the subject's solution of the problem, the development of perception by contrast was completely excluded, although he passed through all stages of adaptation to adequate reading except this one.

We thus find that the set definitely appears in experiments dealing with qualitative problems, and that in quantitative experiments, which involve phenomena of contrast, we are still observing the action of precisely the same set.

Consequently, it may be assumed that the set belongs to the category of facts of reality which may be manifested in the most varied conditions: A set to the values of "greater" or "smaller," or, in general, quantitative relationships of this type, can be produced everywhere that these relationships exist, just as can a set to qualitative attributes.

II. THE METHOD OF STUDY OF THE SET

We have concluded that the illusions described above are based on a certain specific state best described as the set of an actively reacting subject: All these illusions are illusions of the set.

However, if we accept this, we must face a more general problem, not just that of finding the reasons for a specific group of mental phenomena — illusory experience — but the problem of the psychology of the set itself. Accordingly, the whole subsequent text will be devoted to this problem. One of the more important tasks awaiting our attention at the present time is the establishment of our method of investigation.

In the previous pages, we discussed experiments which brought to light several variants of illusions of the set. The question now arises whether we can use the same method for a more complete study of the problem of the set in general.

In the first place, it must be remembered that the problem we are discussing is not an isolated psychological fact, but a specific state which I call the set. As we shall see below, two elementary conditions must be satisfied before this state can develop — some actual demand must be placed on the subject and a situation provided for its satisfaction. If both these conditions are present, the subject will develop a set toward a definite activity. The particular state of consciousness, or its particular manifestation, will arise only on the basis of this set. Consequently, we must draw a strict line between, on the one hand, the set and, on the other, the concrete state of consciousness developing from it. The set itself, of course, is no part of this state, and it is clearly impossible to describe it in terms of the phenomena of consciousness. However, let us assume that we have fixed a set sufficiently firmly. In this case, it will always be represented in consciousness by a particular impression arising on the basis of this set. If this set is repeatedly activated, we shall notice that each time the same impression arises in our consciousness.

Let us now instruct a subject with such a fixed set to experience, or perceive, something only slightly different from what he usually experiences on the basis of this set. What happens in this case? We know from our experiments that this type of situation, besides evoking a new and adequate set, is always experienced on the basis of the existing fixed set. Consequently, we may say that one and the same fixed set may lie at the basis of the identical perception of several different, but closely related, objective situations. The set in this case is responsible for the identification of a group of comparatively similar situations among the experiences. In our experiments, this is expressed by the usual appearance in our critical presentations of the illusory perception of two equal stimuli (for example, balls of equal size) as unequal, which persists for a longer or shorter time, until the fixed set has been suppressed and a new one, adequate to the situation, has had the opportunity to develop.

While this illusory perception is present, we are justified in assuming that the fixed set is active, and, depending on the course of this experience, we may be in a position to judge the properties of this set and to study the course of its development.

We thus see that the observation of illusion provides the opportunity for the study of sets lying at the basis of these experiences. Admittedly, these sets may be only fixed, but, first, it is these which are of particular interest to us, for they are the common basis of human experience, and, second, they contain nothing essentially new in comparison with the actual sets arising on the basis of the subject's new situations and demands, so that to some extent they can also be used to study these actual sets.

III. SOME DOGMATIC POSTULATES OF TRADITIONAL PSYCHOLOGY

Before turning to the investigation of the set, let us first discuss the dogmatic assumptions of traditional psychology which have prevented consideration of this concept. We refer, first, to the problem of the direct link between conscious mental phenomena and, second, to the problem of the character of this link as seen by the empiricists.

1. The Postulate of Spontaneity

It seems to me that modern bourgeois psychology is entirely based on a dogmatically perceived postulate, not previously verified and not susceptible to criticism, according to which objective reality spontaneously and immediately influences the conscious mind and, by this spontaneous link, determines its activity. From this postulate arises a series of ungrounded, spurious problems and fruitless attempts at their solution.

Let us examine more closely this dogmatic postulate of traditional psychology.

The rapid and productive development of the natural sciences has, among other things, largely contributed to the fact that, from the very beginning in this field, the view has been held which was later formulated by some scientists as the principle of "closed causality."

In this particular case, the meaning of this principle lies in the assumption that a physical consequence may be provoked only by the action of a physical cause, that there is a direct or spontaneous link between them, and that for one to act on the other there is no need to seek as an intermediate link any other phenomenon which cannot be placed in the category of physical phenomena. It must be assumed that the comparatively rapid development of the natural sciences in our period would have been quite impossible without the confident belief that physical phenomena are directly related to one another and are determined in the process of this mutual relationship.

Hence, the rapid progress in the natural sciences is largely based on recognition of the direct connection between physical phenomena. It is not surprising, therefore, that the same principle of direct association of phenomena was borrowed by the other sciences in the hope that this would lay the foundations for their equally rapid development.

Obviously, however, the phenomena of mental life make the principle of their direct association difficult to accept.

The purpose of mental processes is to mediate for us the attributes of the external situation, which itself is not a part of mental reality. Despite this, psychologists have attempted to base investigations on the principle of the direct association of phenomena — the direct association between mental phenomena themselves. According to this point of view, mental phenomena have mental causes, and it is within the realm of the mind that explanations for its activity must be sought.

The theoretical basis of this point of view has been given in accordance with the principle of the "closed causality of nature" formulated by Wundt.

Wundt postulated that mental consequences are based on the activity of mental causes. In fact, however, this point of view had been expressed in science even before his time. Herbart, for example, attempted to explain the whole of mental life, the whole of its content, in terms of interaction between ideas. Herbart's view was that these interactions are purely mechanical in character: A strong idea overcomes a weaker one and expels it from the limits of consciousness. Hence, the condition of the mind at any particular moment is entirely dependent on the relationships between the intensity of the ideas present at that moment in the individual. Clearly, Herbart was concerned with the mechanics of ideas.

The principle of spontaneity is perhaps even more clearly defined in the theories of so-called associationist psychology. According to the fundamental postulates of this school, the whole of mental activity is determined by the direct association between ideas: No sooner does one link of this association appear in consciousness than it is followed by the appearance of another idea, associated with it in some sense. Hence, it is clear that, to the associationists, the whole of mental activity is based on associations established between mental phenomena — mental consequences arise on the basis of mental causes; mental processes and phenomena act upon the mental sphere of reality.

Wundt, who was opposed both to Herbart's psychology and to associationist psychology, not only continued to base his views on the principles of spontaneity, but even attempted to give them philosophical foundations. He postulated that the only certain observation which is possible in man is observation of the unity of consciousness, that is, the direct link between psychological phenomena; mental processes themselves are associated with each other and have direct, mutual effects on each other. As an empirical science, psychology must, in Wundt's opinion, be based entirely on these indisputable facts and it must attempt to explain the phenomena with which it is concerned on the basis of these facts; that is, it must explain phenomena of the mind in terms of causes of a mental character. In brief, it must attempt to explain mental facts entirely within the framework of mental life. Any attempt to overstep these limits in order to seek an explanation of mental phenomena outside them must be regarded, according to Wundt, as unscientific and therefore unproductive. Consequently, Wundt believed that the mind must be regarded as the sum of conscious phenomena, mutually associated and acting on each other in accordance with regular principles.

Essentially the same point of view still remains in force in bourgeois psychology at the present time. One of the most influential modern psychological theories, the gestalt theory, emphatically insists on the same principle of the direct interconnection of mental phenomena. The main postulate of this psychological theory is as follows: In the realm of our experiences, integral processes influence each other and thus unite to form complex experiences, and, conversely, these complex experiences determine the realm of individual mental processes taking place in our consciousness. Yet these two processes, both complex and integral or partial and individual, constitute the world of mental phenomena, and consequently, the problem of mental causality is solved, according to the gestalt theory, precisely on the basis of recognition of the idea of a direct interconnection between conscious mental processes. As we see, the idea that conscious mental phenomena are directly associated remains in force.

However, there is another school of thought in modern psychology which does not recognize the principle of psychophysical parallelism, the basic principle of the above-mentioned theories, but rather assumes that interaction between physical and mental phenomena may take place. According to this theory, there is nothing to prevent us from concluding that a causal link may also exist between these two categories of phenomena: The physical, by acting on the mental, gives rise to various processes, and vice versa.

However, the view that a direct connection exists also remains in this case. Here it is assumed that a direct connection exists even between such widely different phenomena as physical and mental. The so-called interactionist theories differ from the parallelistic theories, not in any fundamental principle, but merely in matters of secondary importance; the idea of the direct character of the relationship between these phenomena remains a dogmatically accepted postulate in both these theories.

It is generally accepted, however, that man, like everything living in general, attains the degree of his development appropriate to each given moment only during the process of interaction with the environment. However, from the point of view of the theory of direct causation, this assertion does not reflect the true state of affairs. On the contrary, it supposes that in fact it is not man, but his mind which interacts with the environment, that the mind is the controlling force, and that in essence the whole history of man is created by his mind. This purely idealistic assertion is quite characteristic of the whole of bourgeois psychology, and it is interesting that it is numbered among its cardinal principles.

This attempt to ignore the subject completely and to construct the science of human mental life without any reference to the subject, as was done in traditional psychology, could not of course remain unnoticed even by bourgeois thinkers. In fact, Hegel considered this question in detail and attempted to solve it as best he could. He asserted that the individual is essentially "consciousness or self-awareness" and nothing more. Hence, when discussing the interrelationship of the mind and the external environment, he was essentially trying to say that the subject of these relationships is man, for man is nothing more than "consciousness or self-awareness."

Wundt also attempted to solve this problem in the same light. He asserts that from the point of view of scientific psychology, the subject is merely the sum of his mental functions. To think of a subject in any other light would mean, in his opinion, restoring to science the old concept of substance, which has never made any contribution to progress in the scientific study of the facts of mental life. Hence, we see that Wundt also formulated his attitude to this problem from the standpoint of idealistic philosophy.

The position adopted by Stern is of the greatest interest from the point of view of the problem under consideration. The principles of his "personalistic" psychology are difficult to reconcile with attempts to reduce the concept of the persona — the fundamental concept of his philosophical and psychological theories — with the idea of the sum of the mental facts. Nevertheless, despite many digressions, he was ultimately forced to turn to the idea of a connection between mental processes regulated by the persona. Since his theory gives no precise indications of the reality of anything other than the ordinary mental phenomena which could serve for giving substance to the concept of the persona, he was compelled to restrict himself to these phenomena, apart from the addition of supplementary definitions taken exclusively from a storehouse of metaphysical concepts completely devoid of scientific value. Because of the absence of a positive meaning of the concept of personality in Stern's system, he was compelled to restrict himself to ordinary psychological concepts for his definition.

Hence, it is clear that the generally accepted principle of traditional psychology is the principle of the direct character of the relationship between ordinary mental processes or between mental and physical processes.

2. The Postulate of Empiricism

Among the equally unverified postulates of empirical psychology is the hypothesis that human life must be based on a purely empiricist principle regulating the whole life and behavior of the living being. This principle of empiricism is essentially as follows: The living organism and the environment are separated by a deep abyss which prevents the organism from making direct use of the data presented by this environment. Before the living being can find in the environment something which it requires to satisfy its demands, it must make a series of "trials and errors," continuing this until it accidentally hits on something suitable. The whole life history of such an animal must be like, for example, the behavior of a rat in an experimental maze, which usually finds its bearings in just such a manner. From this point of view, the environment in which the animal lives may be thought of as an enormous maze in which the way can be found only through a large number of trials accompanied by an equally large number of errors. The conditions and mode of life of animals at particular stages of their development are the product of a long series of "trials and errors," following equally long series performed by previous generations.

Such is the basis of the contemporary bourgeois empiricist psychology. It would not be difficult to show how dominant this point of view is in contemporary science. However, I do not wish to dwell on this matter here. I merely wish to draw the reader's attention to the fact that an attempt has recently been made to reduce the dominance of this postulate of empiricism in psychology. I refer to the view held by followers of the gestalt theory regarding the special form of perception of the outside world which they call "insight." This concept is discussed at great length by Köhler, who apparently first introduced it into science. He reports the presence of this method of perception in chimpanzees required to solve a specially devised problem concerned with the seizing of food within their field of vision. The chimpanzees immediately grasped the problem and, after a few unsuccessful experiments, solved it "once and for all," without making gradually more successful attempts. In Köhler's opinion, in this case we are not dealing with a process in which the animal gradually comes nearer to success in solving the problem, but with the fact of the immediate discovery of its solution. He considers that the animal solved the problem by "insight," a different method than the discursive thinking characteristic of man.

Köhler makes no serious attempt to give a more exact definition of insight which would reveal its true nature, and in his subsequent investigations of this problem nothing important is added which could provide a basis for the concept of a unique "mode of thought." Nowadays, therefore, attempts are being made in psychology to define insight as simply a phenomenon of ordinary perceptual processes.

In the present state of modern psychology, there is, of course, nothing unexpected about this conclusion regarding the nature of insight. Since in Köhler's time psychology was limited to concepts dealing with the ordinary phenomena of consciousness, in this case the ordinary perceptual processes unrelated to insight, it is difficult to imagine that his observations could have been adequate to establish a radically new concept.

But if we accept that in addition to the ordinary phenomena of consciousness, we have something else which although not a part of consciousness nevertheless determines it to a considerable degree, we are then in a position to judge phenomena resembling insight from a new point of view; we are in a position to justify the presence of this "something else" and, what is particularly important, to discover something of its real essence.

If we assume that the living being possesses the power to react in certain conditions by activation of the set, if we assume that it is in this set that we shall find the new area of specialized reflection of reality, as we shall discuss in more detail below, then it becomes apparent that it is in this direction that we must seek the key to the understanding of the actual relationship between the organism and the environment in which it must live.

IV. FUNDAMENTAL CONDITIONS OF ACTIVITY

We must begin by defining the two main conditions without which the behavioral acts of man or any other living creature whatever would be impossible. The first of these is the presence of some form of need for the subject to act, and the second is the presence of a situation in which this need may be satisfied. These are the basic conditions for the appearance of any type of behavior and, above all, of a set in relation to it. We must take a closer look at these conditions.

1. The Need

The term "need" is frequently encountered in science. It is used particularly often in the economic sciences. Here, however, we are not thinking only of the special meaning which it assumes in economics, but rather with its broader meaning. If we imagine that an organism experiences a want of something, for example, economic goods or some other object of value — whether practical or theoretical is immaterial — of activity or, conversely, of rest, etc., then in all these instances we can say that we are dealing with some form of need. Briefly, want may be defined as any state of the psychophysical organism which, requiring changes in the surrounding medium, gives impulse to the activity required for this purpose.

It must be remembered here that the term "activity" must be understood not merely as that which provides the means for satisfying needs, but also as the source of their direct satisfaction.

This means that we must distinguish two basic types of needs — substantive needs and functional needs.

The former require something substantial for their satisfaction. Hunger is an example of a particular substantive need: In order to satisfy hunger, we must have food.

However, this not the only category of needs. As we have just mentioned, the organism may experience a desire for some form of activity. The organism in this instance has no need of anything substantial, merely a desire for activity as such, the need is simply for activity. This means that the natural state of the living organism is not immobility. On the contrary, the living organism is in a state of continuous mobility. This state is interrupted only temporarily and in certain conditions — namely, when the organism is in need of rest, though even here there is never an absolute cessation of activity: The organic processes in these cases, as in all other cases, continue to be active. Depending on the conditions in which the organism has to live at each given moment, it may develop a need for activity, a need for function in a certain direction. Needs of this type we call "functional."*

These two main groups constitute the whole of the wide range of needs present in animals. However, they cannot be used as the main categories of the needs appearing in man during the develop-

*D. N. Uznadze, The Psychology of the Child, 1946.

ment of the conditions of his social and cultural life. Culture produces new needs, and the further it develops, the more extensive the range of man's needs. As an example of a need which may be regarded as purely human, we may mention an abstract intellectual need. Admittedly, instances are frequently discussed in the literature when what I call purely human manifestations such as inquisitiveness may be seen in animals, especially in monkeys. Strictly speaking, however, there are no grounds for considering the behavior of even the higher monkeys in anthropomorphic terms. I merely wish to say here that a group of abstract intellectual needs can undoubtedly be distinguished as a specific group of needs arising in man.

But are these needs something new from the point of view of the fundamental classification which we have given above? Can the intellectual need be regarded as substantive or functional?

If we consider the concept of the intellectual need, we find that we are discussing instances where a subject, confronted with the hypothetical solution of a problem, pauses, stops the manipulations which he is carrying out in the process of working on the problem, and converts the problem into an object of special reflection. This is truly the moment of objectivation (which we shall discuss again below), after which the application of intellectual processes to the problem begins [77].

What is the issue here? Into which category can we place the need which we are trying to satisfy in this case?

There is little justification for speaking of functional needs in this case. Abstract intellectual thinking is certainly not directed toward the satisfaction of any functional need. These acts are necessary for definite purposes, let us say for determining the true nature of a problem, or what rules are best to apply in solving it. The problem of the theoretical approach to an object is undoubtedly much closer to the category of substantive needs than to the category of functional needs. During the solution of problems in the latter category, there is no real need for intellectual work: The need does not require processes of realization, frequently essential when substantive needs are to be satisfied. There is nothing surprising about this, for during the satisfaction of substantive needs the problem may always arise of how and to what degree the given material satisfies the present need. This, of course, is a problem which must be realized in the abstract plane before a practical solution can be obtained.

Hence, intellectual needs arise essentially only in the aid of our substantive needs. Since they are always calculated to ensure satisfaction of these substantive needs, we could say that intellectual needs are essentially nothing more than a further complication of substantive needs. Without touching here on the higher degrees of development of the intellect, we can say that, at least in the initial stages of its development, this is nothing more than a form of further complication of the process of satisfaction of substantive needs.

Admittedly, we know that many acts are directed toward the satisfaction of functional needs. However, this is usually only in the presence of obstacles preventing us from performing the necessary acts for satisfaction of these needs. The problem arising in this case — establishing the cause of the difficulties — is not at all functional in character. It is a separate problem, which must be solved in the interest of the subject motivated to satisfy functional needs, but not directly — only indirectly, as an essential condition for achieving his direct purposes.

In brief, in this particular instance we are concerned with a situation in which the achievement of a subject's direct goal — the satisfaction of his functional demands — requires the preliminary solution of an intellectual problem — the elucidation of the causes interfering with the achieving of this goal.

Hence, needs of an intellectual character may also be present in the course of satisfaction of functional needs, but this in no way converts them into functional needs.

It can thus be seen that one of the fundamental conditions for the activity of an individual is the presence in him of a definite need, which may be substantive or functional. At the human level of development we witness the emergence of a new type of need, that is, the intellectual need. Analysis shows, however, that this is essentially more closely related to the category of the substantive needs than to that of the functional.

2. The Situation

Besides the need, the other essential condition for the appearance of a set in a certain direction is the presence of a corresponding situation. If no such situation is present, there is no set; without the presence of the combined and harmonious action of the situation and need on the subject, there is no basis for formation of the set or, consequently, for the subject to be made ready for action.

Naturally, a need may exist in the absence of a situation permitting its satisfaction. In this case, however, it will not have a final, individually determined character. It obtains this only when the existing situation is capable of bringing it satisfaction: The need becomes concrete and individually determined and its satisfaction is possible in the concrete conditions of a given situation only when circumstances allow it. If this situation is not present, the need will remain unindividualized. As soon as definite necessary conditions for the satisfaction of this need appear, however, a concrete set is produced in the subject, and he feels the impulse toward activity in a certain direction. Hence, for a set to develop, it is essential that a corresponding situation be present, in which it assumes a definite, concrete character. Consequently, a situation of this type must be regarded as an objective factor determining the set.

It is clear that creation of the set does not occur as a result of the presence of the need alone or of the objective situation alone: For a set toward definite activity to develop, the need must be combined with a situation embracing the conditions for its satisfaction.

It is interesting here to consider Lewin's theory of the "determining tendency" of a particular group of ideas (Aufforderungscharakter). This determining tendency develops, in his opinion, from our attitude to things and phenomena which we need. When we develop a certain need, the objects or phenomena related to it acquire a certain strength with respect to the need; they compel us to act in a certain direction and stimulate us to carry out certain acts: Bread compels the starving person to seize it and eat it, a bed invites a tired person to lie on it. However, this "tendency," this motivating force, is found only when the subject has a corresponding need. As soon as the need is satisfied, the object and phenomena lose this force.

Lewin's theory is interesting because it stems from the correct observation that objects and phenomena which are a part of the situation providing satisfaction of a real need apparently exert a force over the subject with this need: They literally draw him into it. However, this happens only when the relevant need is present in the subject. In this case, Lewin gives a factual observation which corresponds to the hypothesis of the development of the set in a certain direction only in a subject having a definite need, and in the presence of the situation essential for its satisfaction.

Hence, we see that for a set to develop in a certain direction, conditions of a subjective and objective character are required; both the need and the situation in which it may be satisfied must be present.

These are the two main conditions which are absolutely essential before any definite set can arise. Of course, in the absence of subjective and objective conditions in general, there can be no activity. However, here we are saying more than this; we are also stressing the fact that an essential and necessary condition for the development of the set is the unity of these two conditions. In our case this unity takes place as follows: A need present in a subject becomes a definite concrete need only after an objective situation appears in the form of the concrete situation enabling the subject to satisfy the particular need. Both factors – situation and need – are defined as concrete facts and are connected with each other.

V. GENERAL CHARACTER OF THE SET

1. The Possibility of Experimental Study of the Organism as a Whole

If we examine all the cases in which, as we stated above, the set plays a part, we see that hardly any substantial sphere of relationship between the subject and the outside world exists in which there is no such participation. We establish relationships with the outside world in the first place through our receptors, and those of greatest importance to us are, of course, the distance receptors, that is, the receptors primarily responsible for our visual and auditory impressions. The illusions of objects and the illusions of hearing described above are related to this category of receptors.

The action of the set is also dependent on the so-called concrete or direct receptors, and primarily on the receptors of tactile and muscular sensation. Illusions of orientation, as we have seen, are related to these sensory modalities. The first of these are Müller's illusions of weight, followed by the tactile illusions which I have described. So far as the remaining contact senses – taste and smell – are concerned, similar illusions could be described in relation to these, but since they play a comparatively small role in human relationships to the outside world, we shall not discuss them in detail in this book.

This by no means exhausts the field of application of our illusions. They are not confined to the evaluation of quantitative and qualitative relationships. This becomes clear from a consideration of our experiments with an unfamiliar alphabet, which we mentioned above.

But what does this tell us? If we consider that our illusions may, in certain conditions, arise in all modalities of the human senses, this means that these illusions are general in character and are in no sense illusions brought about by specific conditions of the activity of one particular organ; on the contrary, they are rather illusions rooted in the principles governing the activity of the organism as a whole. In brief, we must assume that these illusions embody one of the principles of activity of the living organism as a single, indivisible whole.

From this point of view, there is no doubt that in these illusions we are dealing with phenomena of much greater importance than any of the other phenomena characterizing the living organism. Experiments with these illusions of the set make feasible, for the first time, the possibility of studying the activity of the living organism as a whole.

2. Irradiation of the Set

If we look deeper into the phenomena of illusions, we see that they must not be thought of as local phenomena. Admittedly, Müller, and after him Ach, as in general all modern psychologists who have stated their views regarding the set, interpret it as one of the ordinary mental processes. However, a more careful investigation of these phenomena, as we shall see below, demonstates conclusively that this point of view is obsolete, and that in the phenomena of the set we are undoubtedly concerned with a new sphere of reality, the study of which is of considerable interest for the understanding of mental life as a whole.

Special experiments which we carried out to study this problem fully confirmed this conclusion.

These experiments were based on the following consideration: Assuming that the set is an ordinary, local process, taking place somewhere in the psychophysical being, it obviously must be related exclusively to those spheres which play a direct part in the fixing experiment, whereas its other spheres must remain completely unaffected. For example, if the set is activated in one hand or one eye, the other member of the pair must remain completely free from its influence. Consequently, in order to activate a set in them also, special fixing experiments must be carried out. But if it is found that the performance of fixing experiments in the region of one eye or one hand is enough to cause the appearance of a set simultaneously in the other member of the pair, this would be an argument in favor of the suggestion that the set is an integral process rather than a narrowly localized one.

This problem was first solved negatively by the experiments of Stephens. This author found that a motor set, which he studied, is a purely local phenomenon, and that if such a set is produced in one hand, it remains there and does not spread to the other member of the pair. The same conclusion was evidently reached by Ach, for when discussing the need for recognizing a specific type of set, what he called the "sensory set," he stressed that the motor set does not spread to the corresponding organ, which could not, in his opinion, be said about the sensory set. Stephens suggested that the set must be understood as a peripheral process, so that there is nothing surprising in the fact that it is limited to the region where it has been specially produced and does not spread mechanically from one organ to another.

Originally, when we were just beginning our investigations of illusions of the set, we verified the accuracy of our experimental results twice for the following reason: At first, during the usual sequence of our investigations, we carried out experiments to study irradiation of the set to the corresponding organ: Fixing experiments were carried out on one hand, let us say the right hand; into the left hand we placed equal balls as critical objects. The results of these experiments, summarized in Table VI, showed unequivocably that the set spreads from one organ to another of its own accord — without any special critical experiments. The number of illusory perceptions in this case was more than 83% in the left hand (Table VI), of which 60% were illusions of contrast.

Hence, this showed conclusively that the motor set, fixed in one of a pair of corresponding organs, spreads automatically to the other organ.

TABLE VI

Number of experiments	+	−	=
85	60%	23.5%	16.5%

TABLE VII

Order of experiments	+	−	=
From right to left	56%	32%	12%
From left to right	64%	24%	12%

We did not learn of the work of Stephens and Ach until much later, and it led us to repeat these experiments in order to verify the accuracy of our results as given in Table VI. At my instruction, the experiments were carried out by one of my colleagues, and the results obtained are given in Table VII. In this case, we see that our experiments were not restricted to transfer of the set from one hand to the other, but included both possible cases – possibility of irradiation from the right hand to the left or from the left to the right. The table shows that the results of these control experiments fully confirmed the accuracy of the results given in Table VI.

In the first place, it is interesting to note that the number of illusory perceptions in both critical experiments was the same: During irradiation both to left and to right it was 88%. The only difference here concerned the distribution of contrast and assimilative illusions.

Still more interesting, however, is the fact that these results agree almost completely with those given in Table VI. This is particularly true of the number most characteristic in these experiments – the number of contrast illusions. In any case, the results of the experiments fully confirmed our hypothesis concerning irradiation of the set from one of a pair of corresponding organs to the other, in this case from one hand to the other.

In our subsequent work, we regarded this problem of the possibility of irradiation of the set from one organ to another as finally solved, and we have not returned to it again. We carry out experiments only to study the degree of irradiation of the set in each individual case.

It must be remembered, however, that the property of irradiation does not characterize the set in any one special modality: It characterizes it in general. From this point of view, we carried out special experiments with different sensory modalities.

In the first place, it had to be established whether a set produced in one eye irradiates to the other eye. For this purpose, we carried out the following variant of our experiment: The subject

TABLE VIII

Number of subjects	+	–	=
86	69.8%	7%	23.2%

closes one (for example, the left) eye and with the other fixes stimuli appearing in a tachystoscope. In fixing experiments, we present two circles of different sizes to him. In the critical experiment, the subject is given two equal circles, and this time he must study them with the left eye and compare them. Thus, these experiments are designed to test whether the set spreads from one eye to the other.

The results of these experiments, given in Table VIII, show that irradiation also takes place in this case. The figure of 76.8% is high enough to demonstrate conclusively that irradiation in the visual sphere undoubtedly occurs.

Hence, we may conclude that a set, fixed in one of paired organs (hand, eye), also irradiates to the other organ, although the latter may evidently be completely excluded from participation in the fixing experiment.

Now, however, a new question arises: Is irradiation of the set confined to the corresponding organs, or can it spread much wider afield? It must be assumed that the answer to this question is positive, if the set is not a local state of some individual part of the organism, but a state of the organism as a whole. For this reason, the results of experiments on this problem must be of considerable interest to us, for they would provide the final solution to the problem with which we are concerned.

A. In one series of experiments, we proceeded as follows: A pair of wooden balls is placed into the subject's hands 15 to 25 times, the larger ball into the right hand and the smaller into the left. After these fixing series, we carry out the critical experiment tachystoscopically; the subject must optically compare the areas of two objectively equal circles. The results of these experiments must solve the problem with which we are concerned here. They must show whether a set created in the haptic sphere can influence the evaluation of relationships of optic perceptions or, expressed more precisely, whether a set fixed in the hands is confined to the region of the hands or whether it may involve the visual region in the sphere of its influence. The results of these experiments, carried out in our laboratory, are shown in Table IX.

TABLE IX

Number of experiments	+	−	=	?
71	48%	8.4%	21.5%	22%

In this instance, we see that our results generally confirm the hypothesis that the set may also irradiate to such remote spheres as the haptic and visual. We find that irradiation occurs in not less than 56.4% of cases. This is a sufficiently high figure to prove beyond doubt that phenomena of this type do occur.

But more evidence is needed. In these experiments, the figures used as critical objects differed from each other by approximately 1 to 2 mm. When, in the fixing experiments, the larger ball is placed in the right hand and the smaller in the left, in the critical experiments the larger (by 1 to 2 mm) circle is shown on the right and the smaller on the left. Despite this, the number of contrast illusions obtained in these conditions amounts to 48% of the total. It must be assumed that this percentage would be considerably increased if the subjects had received equal stimuli, as is the usual practice, in the critical experiments. In any case, there is no doubt that 48% contrast illusions is a figure which shows conclusively that in these conditions the illusion is an established fact.

B. If, however, we consider the problem of whether irradiation can spread in the opposite direction, that is, from the optic to the haptic field, then the series of experiments carried out in our laboratory [4] demonstrates clearly that irradiation is observed here also. Admittedly, the number of decisions that the experimental critical objects were unequal is comparatively low, as usual in irradiation experiments, but at the same time irradiation of the set – in the form of predominance of contrast and assimilative illusions together – is observed in more than 46% of all cases (Table X).

In these experiments, which were carried out by Adamashvili in accordance with my instructions to verify the irradiation of the set in a series of sensory modalities (from haptic to optic, from muscular to haptic, from optic to muscular, and vice versa), the usual experiments were made more precise, in the sense that the subjects were required to concentrate their attention, not on the material with which the experiments were carried out, but only on the correlation of the experimental objects. When this is done, as we have shown, the percentage of illusory perceptions is somewhat

TABLE X

Irradiation	+	−	=	?
From optic to haptic	13.3%	33.3%	26.6%	26.6%
From muscular to haptic	46.6%	6.6%	13.3%	33.3%
From haptic to muscular	13.3%	13.3%	20.0%	53.3%
From optic to muscular	26.6%	6.6%	13.3%	53.3%
From muscular to optic	20.0%	33.3%	26.6%	20.1%

smaller, which probably explains the slight reduction in illusory readings in these experiments. Nevertheless, the percentage is still high enough to show that irradiation of illusions may take place in different directions.

C. Next, it is interesting to learn whether a set fixed in the muscular sphere irradiates into the haptic sphere, and vice versa, and if so, to what degree. The results of experiments carried out especially for this purpose are given in Table X.

We find that the index of irradiation of the set in this instance is relatively high: More than 53% contrast and assimilative illusions together is by no means a low figure. The results become even more convincing if attention is directed to their distribution in the table, especially to the number of contrast illusions, which are most indicative in these quantitative experiments.

D. We next consider the question of irradiation of the set in the opposite direction, from the haptic sphere to the muscular. The same table shows that this also occurs, although in comparatively few cases (26.6% contrast and assimilative illusions together). If, however, we consider the comparatively high percentage of uncertain answers, it is clear that 26.6% illusions in these conditions is quite adequate to prove that irradiation of the set also occurs here, as in the converse experiments in which, as we have just seen, the number of cases of irradiation amounted to over 53%.

E. So far as irradiation of the set from the optic sphere to the muscular is concerned, it is clear that the percentage of uncertain answers here also was very high (53.3%), which of course had an effect on the percentage of irradiated illusions. For example, the total number of cases of irradiation here was 33.2%. Bearing in mind that the number of cases in which no illusions whatever were found was comparatively low (13.3%), then the figure of 33.2%

certain cases of irradiation in these conditions must be interpreted as a reasonably high figure.

F. If, finally, we examine the results concerning irradiation of the set in the opposite direction, from the muscular sphere to the optic, we see that they are on a relatively high level (Table X). The total number of cases of irradiation here was more than 53%, and the number of cases of its absence was comparatively low (26.6%). From this we may conclude that a set, established toward the differentiation of weight, also extends to the optic sphere and determines the perception of objects of equal size as being clearly unequal.

Hence, we see that all these experiments conclusively show that irradiation of the set from one sensory region to another may take place. The impression is gained that the sensory modalities examined here, which have become adequately differentiated in the history of development of the species, have not lost their basic unity; they are still the organs of an integral whole, which uses them as auxiliary tools for the solution of problems placed before it.

3. Generalization of the Set

We must now examine one further property of the set, a property which we have already had occasion to mention above.

We have just seen that one of the fundamental features of the set is its irradiation. Besides this, however, we have discovered one further feature of the set, which evidently lies close to the property of irradiation. I have called this "generalization."

When we produce any form of fixed set in a subject, let us say the set that a ball on the right is smaller than a ball on the left, we find in critical experiments that this set remains in force when applied to various other objects having little in common with a ball, for example, in relation to cubes, to polygons, and so on. The action of the set is seen more clearly still in tachystoscopic experiments in which the shapes can be varied much more easily than in the critical experiments.

Above, when we were discussing the factor of the figure in the action of the set, we encountered findings related to those which we are now examining.*

*Z. I. Khodzhava, Action of the Set on the Basis of Abstraction of Material, Tr. Gos. Univ. 17:51-100 (1941). N. L. Eliava, The Process of Cessation of the Action of a Set Established to a Pure Correlation, Tr. Gos. Univ. 17:197-206 (1941).

We say then that a set fixed, for example, on the difference in area between two circles assimilates a series of critical figures having very little in common with a circle. As we know, this may go so far that we can say that the set in these cases is fixed more on the correlation as a whole than on the correlation between the particular figures.

4. The "Extraconscious" Nature of the Set

We have shown that the set, as it concerns material received by a subject by means of all his receptor organs, must be understood not as their special functions but as a general state of the individual. The facts of its wide irradiation and generalization, which we have just discussed, confirm and define this statement.

The question then arises: How can we understand this state? If the set is a phenomenon of consciousness, then it must be regarded as one of many such phenomena. However, we have seen that the set cannot be placed in this category. It must rather be regarded as a general state, which concerns not the individual organs of a subject, but his activity as a whole.

Facts pertaining to this question can best be obtained experimentally. We have had previous occasion to use experiments with posthypnotic suggestion [70] to solve problems concerning the theory of expectation as the basis of illusions of the set. We assume that the same experiments can provide us with a definite answer to this new problem.

We have already described how these experiments are carried out. After the subject has been brought into a state of deep hypnotic sleep, balls are placed into his hands, one large and the other small, and he is instructed to compare them and to say which is the larger. After many repetitions of these experiments, the subject recovers from his hypnotic state in another room, where the critical experiments are carried out, when equal balls are placed into his hands and he is asked to compare them.

We have already discussed these experiments in another context. However, the results obtained are also of considerable interest from the present point of view.

The subjects, who know nothing of the fixing experiments carried out during hypnotic sleep, nevertheless exhibit the usual illusion of the set in the critical experiment: One of the balls nearly always appears to be larger than the other, and this is determined by the influence of the fixing experiments carried out during hypnotic sleep. It must be noted that, as mentioned above, despite the fact of the usual posthypnotic amnesia, we nevertheless suggested to the subjects that they would not remember what they had done during hypnotic sleep. This undoubtedly means that the subjects, although they remember nothing consciously of the fixing experiments performed during hypnotic sleep, nevertheless are actually under the determining influence of these experiments.

It is perfectly clear that, as a result of the fixing experiments, they develop some form of state which, while remaining outside their consciousness, still exerts a decisive influence on it; if no fixing experiments were carried out with them, as a rule they perceived the equal balls of the critical experiments quite adequately.

Hence, it can be concluded that a state may exist which, although not a part of consciousness, has the power to act decisively upon it. In our experiments, this state is produced as a result of the action of fixing experiments, and the fact that equal critical balls are perceived as unequal is the logical result of the activity of this "extraconscious" state.

In brief, we may conclude from the results of these experiments that conscious states may be under the influence of other processes which are not necessarily conscious; they may also be determined by processes which have no definite place in consciousness and which, therefore, are not conscious mental facts. As our experiments conclusively show, in addition to conscious mental processes, what may be called "extraconscious" processes may also exist, although this feature does not prevent them from playing a very important role. This role, as we have seen, is here played by the set, which we have previously fixed in our subjects during hypnotic sleep. This set, in our experiments, was never a part of consciousness. Nevertheless, it undoubtedly had the power to act upon it; objectively equal balls were perceived as quite definitely unequal.

Hence, we may conclude that conscious experiences may take place under the definite influence of the set, which for its part is not a component of consciousness.

5. Superfluity of the Concept of the Unconscious

We may accordingly assume that the widespread theories concerning the important role of the unconscious in human mental activity undoubtedly rest on a very firm basis. However, closer acquaintance with these theories shows that this basis is not very well understood, so that the whole concept of what the unconscious is becomes unconvincing and excessively artificial.

There is no doubt that the weakest point in the theory of the unconscious, for instance, as understood by Freud, is the assertion that conscious and unconscious processes are fundamentally identical, although by definition the former is accompanied by consciousness, while the latter is not. So far as the two processes are concerned, their internal nature and structure are the same, although they differ externally.

In the light of this interpretation, it can be understood that unconscious processes, which play so important a role, for example, in mental diseases, may be made conscious, at first with the assistance of the psychoanalyst, and later, in certain conditions, by the patient himself. According to the psychoanalysts, no new or fundamental change takes place in the patient's mind as a result of his experiences: Before, nothing of its content was illuminated by the rays of consciousness, but once it is illuminated this is basically enough to make the patient healthy.

According to this theory, everything depends on the patient's past life — on experiences which were or might have been conscious, but in the first instance were rejected into oblivion, and in the second were expelled from consciousness from the very beginning. "To realize" in this context means nothing more than "to recollect." It seems as though forgotten elements of consciousness continue to live and act outside consciousness, and thus exert their influence on the subject's behavior.

The most important source of difficulty in, for example, the theory of Freud is this concept of the unconscious. I think that if we could establish that the mental content of the unconscious is not that usually associated with conscious life but still not radically separated from it, we would possess a weapon which would enable us to obtain a much deeper understanding of the true state of affairs.

We have seen that the concept of the set is in fact the most suitable for solving this problem. The set — as we have seen in experiments with posthypnotic suggestion — is a state which, although not an element of consciousness, nevertheless has a decisive influence on its working. In this case, the present state of affairs would be imagined as follows: Our ideas and thoughts, our senses and emotions, our voluntary decisions are elements of our conscious mental life, and when these mental processes begin to appear and to act, they are necessarily accompanied by consciousness. To be conscious, therefore, means to imagine and to think, to experience emotions, and to perform acts of volition. Consciousness has no other meaning than this. But it would be wrong to assert that this exhausts the characteristics of the living organism in general, and of man in particular, aside from his physical being. Besides his conscious processes, something goes on which is not an element of consciousness, but which largely determines it, which lies, so to speak, at the basis of these conscious processes. We have found that this is the set, which actually appears in any living being in the course of its interaction with the outside world. We have seen from our experiments that it actually exists, without assuming the form of an element of consciousness: It actually takes place outside consciousness, but nevertheless it has a decisive influence on the whole of mental life.

We thus find that the theory of the unconscious is only partly based on a correct interpretation of the mind. It rightly stresses that conscious processes are by no means the whole of the mind, and that therefore we must recognize processes taking place outside consciousness. We can see that the concept of the set, as defined in our hypnotic experiments, suits this situation admirably.

This leads to the conclusion that, without the participation of the set, no mental processes in general, as conscious phenomena, exist, and that before consciousness could begin to work in a particular direction, it was necessary to have activation of a set, determining its direction in each individual case.

VI. VARIANTS OF THE STATE OF THE SET

1. The Fixed Set

In the presence of a need which must be satisfied and an appropriate situation, the living organism resorts to a definite, goal-directed activity. However, as we have shown, this activity arises in the first place in the form of a set, which later develops in the form of internal and external behavioral acts which can be observed. We must now consider the question of how and in what forms this process of creation of the set takes place.

In our experiments, we generally begin with a series of presentations of experimental objects (fixing experiments), after which we move on to the critical presentations and show how the preceding fixing experiments influence them.

What is the role of these fixing experiments? We discussed above the phenomenon of fixation, the result of the repeated presentation of these experiments to the subject. We consider that as a result of the frequent repetition of these experiments, the set arising in response to each separate presentation becomes fixed in the subject. It is the repetition which is the decisive factor in enabling the set arising during each presentation to become fixed. These repeated preliminary experiments have therefore been called "fixing experiments."

The possibility that repetition here played the role of a factor acting in conjunction with the process of fixing is another question which we shall not discuss here. We may note simply that a single presentation of the fixing objects was usually inadequate to ensure that the set corresponding to this exposure remained dominant in the subject to the extent that subsequently presented equal objects were perceived in accordance with it, and consequently appeared unequal. For this reason, the number of presentations must be increased in order to provide an adequately fixed set.

Fixation of the set may also take place in the following conditions: Let us suppose that in response to a certain situation I develop a corresponding set which plays its role by influencing my behavior and then ceases to act. What happens to it thereafter? Does it disappear completely without trace, as if it had never existed, or does it continue to exist in some way, still capable of exerting some influence on my behavior?

If the experimental conclusion described above is correct, that the set is an integral modification of the personality or the subject in general, then there is no doubt that, having played its role, the set must immediately give way to another new set to determine the next action. But this does not mean that the previous set has gone out of circulation once and for all. On the contrary, should the subject meet the same situation with the same intentions again, then the previous set must return appreciably quicker than a new set would develop in a completely new situation. This suggests that a set, once activated, generally does not disappear, but remains ready to be reactivated, provided that suitable conditions arise.

Clearly, this state of preparedness is not always the same. It must depend to some extent on the degree of stability of the set, as measured by the number of repeated fixing experiments; the more often these experiments are repeated — within the limits of the optimum number for each particular subject — the more firmly the set is fixed and the stronger the power of activation embodied in it.

On the other hand, in our experiments it becomes finally clear that isolated cases exist in which the activity of a set leaves a very considerable trace behind it irrespective of the presence of repetition; sets formed on this basis are fixed regardless of the repetition of the fixing experiment and thus become much more easily activated. In all these cases, the moment a situation similar to the current situation arises, this is adequate to activate the set and to direct the subject accordingly.

We must see that cases exist in which, as a result of frequent repetitions of fixing experiments or of their great personal weight, the set becomes so easily excited that it is activated even in response to inadequate stimuli, thus masking the possible development of an adequate set.

It is of course unnecessary that, during the action of a fixed set, a form of set adequate to the particular situation should always disappear and be replaced by another fixed set that is similar, yet different in some respects. There is nothing to prevent us from assuming that cases may also occur in which a subject would have to deal with a situation completely identical to that in which this particular form of fixed set was produced. In such cases, the activated fixed set would coincide completely with that which must be regarded as adequate in this particular case.

Hence, in ordinary conditions of life, and not in experimental conditions, we find not only cases in which a set adequate to a particular situation is replaced by a similar fixed set, but also cases in which the fixed set is completely identical to the adequate set.

On the other hand, cases may also occur in which the activated sets are not those which were fixed sometime during the life of the particular individual, but during the history of the species. In another context, I have often had to point to the development of activity of this type, for example, during the life of a child — to facts which cannot be said to be due to a need for obtaining whatever it is which results from this activity. In the life of a child it frequently happens that some activity is started entirely because the child develops a strong tendency to do it; the need which is excited is the need to function or to be active. This need, which I call a "functional tendency," must be regarded as an inborn form of fixed set.*

*D. Uznadze, The Psychology of the Child, 1946.

2. The Diffuse Set

However, the preliminary experiments are not necessarily fixing experiments always. Sometimes they play a completely different role. It may occasionally happen that for some form of individually determined set to arise, one presentation of a situation to the subject is adequate. It must be assumed that in the initial stages of development of a new set, its individual features are not immediately defined. A more or less prolonged process is necessary before the set is defined as such, before it is differentiated or identified as a state specifically adequate for the actual conditions of behavior.

Consequently, we assume that when it is produced for the first time, the set is a comparatively undifferentiated, unindividualized state. For it to become differentiated as an adequate set in the particular conditions, repeated presentation of appropriate stimuli is necessary. In such cases, the repetition of the fixing experiments has a quite definite purpose, distinct from that of fixation — it is aimed at the differentiation of the set.

This is particularly necessary for the production of sets which are new and unfamiliar to the subject. When in such cases a new object, seen for the first time, begins to act on the subject, the set which it evokes must be diffuse and ill-defined in character. We may say that it is not sufficiently differentiated and, as a result of this, the subject cannot identify this object precisely. Only with the course of time, as the number of repeated presentations of the same object increases, does the set which it evokes gradually differentiate and become defined as the specific set for the particular situation.

Consequently, the preliminary experiments are not only fixing, but also differentiating.

VII. EXCITABILITY (FIXABILITY) OF THE SET

1. Experiments on the Excitability of the Set

Without discussing the question of the importance in principle of repetition, we will now examine the role of repetition in the process of the fixation and differentiation of the set. As we have discovered, a certain measure, admittedly not precisely but nevertheless firmly established, of repetitions exist which is essential for the fixation of the set in each individual case. If we examine from this point of view the results obtained with different subjects, this gives us adequate material to determine the differences between them in this respect.

Experiments for this purpose are carried out very simply: After comparison of the fixing objects — let us say balls of different sizes — the subject indicates the relationship between the sizes of equal (critical) objects. This is repeated until the subject indicates that they are equal. The number of fixing presentations consequently increases gradually, and this continues until the subjects develop illusions of the inequality of objectively equal critical stimuli. Hence, we can determine how many fixing experiments are necessary before an illusion appears for the first time.

On the basis of data showing the number of fixing experiments required for the development of an illusion, we establish the degree of excitability of the fixed set.

Our experiments show that subjects differ considerably from each other in this respect. In some cases one preliminary fixing experiment is sufficient for critical objects to be perceived in an illusory manner. It may also happen, however, that even a comparatively large number of preliminary exposures is insufficient for this purpose. In brief, the excitability of the fixed set is a property which varies individually and within wide limits.

To determine the minimal number of fixing experiments, all that is necessary is to establish the lower threshold of excitation of the illusion, but this does not mean that the excitability of the fixed set is thereby fully described. A continuation of the same experiments shows that the maximal number of repeated presentations necessary to secure optimal fixation of the set by no means coincides with the threshold numbers of these presentations. In other words, cases may occur when a set for whose initial excitation a few exposures are adequate requires a larger number of preliminary experiments for its optimal fixation, much larger than for minimal fixation.

In brief, the results of these experiments showed that the lower threshold of excitability of the set by no means coincides with the threshold of its optimal excitation. This observation showed conclusively that each threshold of excitation of a fixed set is an independent value, and by determining it we can define the character of subjects from different points of view.

2. The Excitability of the Differentiated Set

The establishment of the degree of excitability of the fixed sets in our subjects does not complete the definition of the set. Besides the concept of fixation, there is another point of view which applies to the set, and if the set is to be defined fully, this cannot be ignored. I refer to the differentiation of the set. Admittedly, its range of application is comparatively narrow; it applies only in the case of incompletely formed sets. However, where these occur, it is of great interest to examine their gradual development toward more complete differentiation. As our many experiments have shown, the results are of undoubted value in the analysis of differentiation in our subjects.

VIII. EXPERIMENTAL EXTINCTION OF THE FIXED SET

The next problem to which we must turn our attention is this: How does the set disappear when special measures other than the time factor are the primary influence in its extinction? We shall see below that the fixed set, protected against the action of the time factor, weakens and ultimately disappears completely, being replaced by another set adequate to the new conditions. This is not the question we are considering now; we are interested in what happens if special measures are taken to extinguish a set fixed in experimental conditions.

1. Experimental Methods

The method used for this purpose is simple. It consists of the repetition of critical exposures until a sufficient number of correct answers is received to the question of their relationship. The first time that the subject describes the objects as equal is naturally not sufficient for the experiment to be regarded as completed. This can only be assumed after equality has been established five times in succession, as we showed some time ago in special investigations of this problem.*

The subject must often follow a long and sometimes complicated path before he reaches the stage of recognizing critical objects as equal. The results of a special investigation of this problem provided a clear picture of the state of affairs [82]. It was

*N. Eliava, Stopping the Action of a Set Produced in Response to a Pure Correlation, Tr. Gos. Univ., Vol. 17 (1941).

found that the process of extinction of a fixed set passes through a number of distinct stages before it reaches the state of complete realization.

What is the course of extinction of the fixed set in the experimental conditions which we described above?

2. Condition of the Fixed Set

In the first place, it must be mentioned that we are dealing with a fixed set to quantitative relationships, mainly to the relationship of "larger" and "smaller." This fact must be borne in mind to avoid falling into error and considering that the results of these experiments have a general significance, extending to all cases of action of the set.

We find that during repeated presentation of critical objects, the subject interprets them as unequal — let us say, the object on the right appears larger than the object on the left. It is interesting that in the fixing experiments, the object placed on the right was always smaller in size than the object on the left. This means that the subject in this case had become the victim of an illusion, which, consequently, may be interpreted as an illusion of contrast.

A. The Phase of Illusions of Contrast

If presentation of the same objects continues, the subject will remain for a short time under the influence of the same contrast illusion. In some cases, the number of these illusions actually reaches the level of a continuous series. We may conclude from a large number of results that if the number of illusions of contrast reaches three or more, in this case we are dealing with the first stage or the first phase of action of the set.

Analysis of the results shows that this stage is found only if a series of contrast illusions is detected from the very beginning. (This has to be pointed out specially because we frequently encounter cases in which the first two or three exposures give no illusions whatever; a series of contrast illusions, which may be quite prolonged, starts only after the third or fourth exposure.) It must be assumed that in this particular case we are dealing with the most stable state of fixation of the set. This initial phase of action of the fixed set is the most stable and persistent.

B. The Phase of Appearance of Assimilative Illusions

Immediately after this first stage follows the second phase of action of the set, characterized by obvious signs of beginning extinction. As a result of a series of repeated presentations of the critical objects, the initial stage of a change in the fixed set becomes apparent; it weakens slightly, so that the subject begins to demonstrate assimilative illusions as well as contrast illusions. In this case, we may assume, we have reached the second phase of regressive development of the set – the phase which essentially begins to show for the first time the fact that a change has occurred into the subsequent state of weakening of the still active fixed set.

This phase of regressive development of the set does not occur in all cases of extinction. It is found most frequently in pathological conditions of the set, but it is also often found in quite healthy individuals.

It frequently happens also that the regressive process, developing gradually, gives rise to a large increase in the number of assimilative illusions. This may proceed to such a degree that the number of assimilations begins to exceed the number of contrast illusions, and the latter gradually become less and less frequent until they disappear completely, so that purely assimilative illusions are found. In ideal cases the whole process can be broken up into a series of separate phases, and as a result we obtain several independent levels of development.

C. The Phase of Perception of Reality

In this stage of development the fixed set continues in an active state – it still makes its presence known by preventing adequate reflection of real objects; the subject remains in the power of the fixed set. This is where we witness the appearance of a new phase in the process of regressive development of the fixed set. The subject begins to remark from time to time that the objects he is examining are not unequal, but equal critical objects. He sees this with increasing frequency until, after a short time, he finally passes into the stage of recognizing their equality. This is a new phase of the regressive development of the fixed set which completes this process.

Theoretically, of course, we may assume the presence of many more stages in the regressive course of development of the set. In practice, however, we usually observe the appearance and replacement of these three phases only.

3. Differentiation of the Types of Fixed Set Depending on the Process of Its Extinction

This does not mean, of course, that extinction of a fixed set may be achieved only as a result of passage through all three phases.

Many instances are known in which a fixed set is extinguished after passing through only one or two of these phases.

Depending on the order and completeness of passage through all these stages of extinction of the set, we may distinguish the following cases [21]:

A. The Static Set: Plastic and Coarse

Among a group of subjects a certain number can be found who, after a given number of fixing experiments, are unable to go beyond the limits of action of the fixed set. However often the critical objects are exposed to them, they do not perceive them as equal. In such case, it may be considered that we are dealing with persons characterized by predominance of immobile, inert, or static forms of set. Admittedly, during the many years of our practical investigation of the set, we have invariably come to the same conclusion concerning the low incidence of this type of individual among normal subjects, but nevertheless they must be regarded as forming an independent type which, as we shall see below, is composed of a group of persons with undoubtedly distinctive characterological features.

However, besides this group we may distinguish another, differing from the first in that they pass through several phases of extinction of the set, but never reach the phase of complete disappearance. This means that the subjects of this group, besides experiencing illusions, sometimes produce absolutely correct answers. In this instance we are dealing with subjects who cannot develop a set which is as stable as that in the preceding group; nevertheless, their set is static to the extent that it does not enable them to reach the ultimate correct assessment of the relationship between the acting stimuli.

Hence, it may be concluded that whereas in the first case we are dealing with persons with a stable, static set, in the second case the set is static, but much less stable.

A particularly characteristic feature of the subjects of the first group is the coarseness of their set. This can be concluded from observations showing that the character of their set, when fixed in the process of preliminary experiments, cannot be changed in any degree whatever by the action of objective agents.

In contrast, among the subjects a second group was found who, although they could not ultimately determine the equality of the objects given to them in critical experiments, nevertheless exhibited some signs of development of the process: At first they gave answers characteristic of the second stage of the process of extinction of the set, and later they sometimes gave answers related to the third stage. This, however, was the end of the matter; no further progress was possible, and the subject could not finally decide that the critical objects were equal.

In this instance the same coarseness of the set which characterizes the first two groups is undoubtedly present—the set here is plastic in character, yet it still remains static.

Hence, the static set can be either plastic or coarse.

B. The Dynamic Set: Plastic and Coarse

The next group of subjects behaves as follows in the critical experiments: At first, we see the usual contrast illusions of the set, followed by occasional cases in which the critical objects are described as equal, and finally the subjects conclude once and for all that they are equal. This means that the set, which was fixed in the process of experiments specially conducted for this purpose, gradually weakens and is superseded by a new set more adequate to the current situation. It must be emphasized in particular that here the adequate situation does not come into force inmediately, but as a result of passing through the consecutive stages of its gradual extinction.

Consequently, we can speak neither of the coarseness of the set nor of its static nature. The set in this case may be described as plastic, since the change to the ultimate decision concerning the relationship between the critical objects does not take place immediately but through a series of stages, and dynamic, since the subject does not stay in one of the preceding stages but moves forward and ultimately decides that the critical objects presented to him are equal.

The erradication of the state produced in the fixing experiment and the creation of a set adequate to these conditions are eventually reached by the two preceding groups of our subjects. However, they do not begin to make an adequate assessment of the critical objects gradually, moving from phase to phase, but directly from the phase from which they begin their series of decisions concerning the relationship between these objects. The characteristic feature of both these groups is that they both reach the stage of recognizing the equality of the critical objects; that is, they both become free from the influence of the fixing experiments. However, they do not do so gradually, moving from one stage to another, but immediately—jumping from the stage where they have been from the beginning directly to deciding that the critical objects are equal. We see that the set in both these groups is dynamic because at the end of the experiments they reveal an adequate set. However, it does not possess plasticity so that it may be defined as a coarse dynamic set.

C. The Unfixable Set

Finally, we may note the presence of a completely distinctive group of subjects who, in contrast to the other groups, never fall under the influence of the fixing experiments, never fix the set which arises in each individual case, and therefore always give the correct estimate of the size of the experimental objects. We see that the usual number of fixing exposures is inadequate for the production of a fixed set in these subjects, so that a new set arises as a result of each individual exposure.

In this case, we may assume that we are dealing with persons lacking in internal directing power, and apparently entirely under the control of outside impressions, and thus distinguished by their extreme extraversion.

IX. EXTINCTION OF THE SET DURING PROLONGED EXPOSURES

1. Experiments with the Prolonged Exposure of Critical Objects

We have seen that the process of extinction of the set in our experimental conditions takes place in a definite order; a series of stages is found through which the fixed set must pass before it disappears completely. However, it is possible that the extinction of the set in this way may only take place in our experimental conditions, and not necessarily in all conditions in which this may happen. In order to verify this, we slightly modified our usual experiments; the order of the fixing experiments remained the same as usual, and only the critical presentations were altered.

Instead of exposing the critical objects for a short time, we left them in the subject's hands or before his eyes for a long time until he finally determined that the objects were equal. The question of the duration of the exposures was studied in special experiments. It was found that the optimal duration of the exposures was less than one minute: in 55% of our subjects the set was extinguished during this time (in 22 of the total number of 40 persons). Longer periods were necessary only for comparatively small numbers of subjects (1 to 2 min for 7.5%, 2 to 3 min for 12.5%, and 4 to 5 min for 10%).

2. The Results of These Experiments*

A. After the subject had received 15 fixing exposures, he took the critical objects which were left in his hands for one minute and described their relationship. The answers were approximately as follows: At first a contrast illusion appeared, and this remained in force for a fairly long time. The objects then began to appear equal, but this stage was passed through quickly, and the subject then said that the ball on the left had become bigger (assimilative illusion). This was followed by another perception of equality, but this quickly disappeared: "now the one on the right has become bigger," and this contrast illusion persisted for a comparatively long time, after which the subject finally decided that the critical balls were equal.

Hence, the subject passed through three definite stages before finally deciding that the objects presented to him were equal—first, a prolonged contrast illusion, followed by a brief impression of equality and a series of assimilative illusions, and finally a series of cases of equality and illusions, after which the fixed set was finally extinguished.

B. Other types of extinction of the fixed set may be found. The second type is represented by the following: At first, a contrast illusion acts for a comparatively long time; perceptions of equality are then interspersed, but the contrast illusion still remains the dominant form of reaction, and, last of all, perceptions of equality begin to predominate, in the course of time becoming the final form of the reaction. In these cases we are dealing with a type which differs from the preceding form only in that the second stage—the stage of assimilative illusions—is completely absent and the whole process is accomplished in two stages—the stage of contrast illusions and the stage of the contrast illusions interspersed with instances of perception of equality.

C. One of the subjects gave the following type of reaction: The circles presented to him appeared unequal (45 sec); at first, the circle on the left appeared much larger, but later, it became smaller and appeared to be almost the same size as the circle on the right. This process ultimately stopped, and the subject remarked that the circles had become equal.

In this instance we are dealing with the gradual loss of contrast in the illusion, followed by its complete disappearance.

*K. Mdivani, The Process of Suppression of the Set in Conditions of Prolonged Exposure, Tr. Gos. Univ. im. Stalina, Vol. 17.

D. Finally, cases of the following type were found: After 15 fixing presentations, an illusion appeared at once and remained unchanged throughout the period of exposure. The remarks made by one of the subjects were as follows: "bigger on the right... on the right... on the right... still on the right, but not so much as before... still the same... again bigger on the right, but only very slightly!... still bigger on the right...." In this instance, the fixed set was not completely extinguished.

Special investigation of the reactions of these subjects to short exposures of the experimental object showed that essentially the picture remained the same in both cases; the subjects gave the same order of succession of the stages of disappearance of the fixed sets in the experiments with prolonged exposure of the critical objects as in the experiments with brief exposure.

The only point to be especially emphasized here is that in the experiments with long exposure it was possible to study what was happening with the experimental objects. In the experiments with short periods of exposure, this was impossible, since the duration of exposure was inadequate.

In the experiments with long exposures of the critical objects, the following results were observed: The subjects were all able to witness the dynamic nature of the processes taking place with the experimental objects. Whereas in the experiments with short exposures of the critical objects as a rule all that was mentioned was the difference in size (the statement was made that one circle or ball was bigger than the other), in the long-exposure experiments, it was often remarked that the objects were changing in size, either "becoming wider" or "becoming narrower." In ordinary short-exposure experiments, the "experiences of transition" (Übergangserlebnis) appeared only very rarely, in exceptional cases, while, in the experiments with prolonged exposures, they became the rule. We give below a few examples of how the subjects experienced these phenomena.

Patient No. 6. "At first the edge on the right became thick. It seemed to swell beyond its normal limit, as if it were opening outward. It gradually became bigger and bigger... and then smaller and smaller. As soon as I looked at it carefully, the circle began to grow smaller and narrower. The longer I looked, the smaller it became ... it seemed to move further away from me. Then the circles became equal."

Replies such as this were frequently found; 62.25% of the subjects observed this process of narrowing of the circle which had at first seemed to them to be larger. They therefore had the impression that the circles were becoming equal in size, finally becoming absolutely equal.

If we now take a closer look at the distribution of the stages through which the subjects passed during these experiments, we see that the picture obtained was basically the same as in the experiments with short exposures. The only feature to attract attention was the comparatively high percentage of results indicating a coarse set (67.5%) and a low percentage indicating a plastic set (32.5%), which was never found in the experiments with short exposures.

A careful analysis of cases indicating a coarse set should help to elucidate this situation. As mentioned above, the subjects often stressed in their replies the presence of an "experience of transition." These experiences show that where we thought we were dealing with forms of coarse sets, in fact we were dealing with a special form of plastic set, which could be called a form of "latent plasticity."*

By this we mean the numerous cases encountered in our experiments in which the subjects described an apparent phenomenon of internal movement in the recognition of the sizes of the critical objects. Briefly, during observations of the phenomena of the coarse set, cases of "experience of transition" were found so often that it could be assumed that a plastic form of set rather than a coarse form was present.

Admittedly, the plasticity in this instance is latent—it comes to light only during observations in experiments with prolonged exposures; nevertheless, there is no doubt about its presence. This is perhaps the special feature of our experiments with prolonged exposures which gives them a specific place among the whole range of methods used to study the set.

Hence, we may conclude that the extinction of the fixed set is a gradual process occupying a definite period of time, not only in experiments with brief exposures of critical objects but also in those in which the objects are presented for long periods.

In order to ascertain conclusively that the extinction of fixed sets is essentially a long-term process, we must examine what happens when this takes place entirely under the influence of prolonged time intervals, that is, when the set itself "dies a natural death" without special outside interference.

*K. D. Mdivani, Op. cit.

X. THE PROCESS OF NATURAL EXTINCTION OF THE FIXED SET

1. Stability of the Fixed Set

It is clear from the preceding section that the fixed set possesses some resistance to attempts to extinguish it, and that the process of extinction takes place only gradually, until after a certain time interval it completely disappears. The question now arises: Is not the disappearance of the fixed set simply the natural result of the fact that special measures were taken for this purpose—the repeated and prolonged exposure of critical stimuli to the subject until the action of the fixed set ceased?

To answer this question, we must investigate the activity of the fixed set at various more or less prolonged time intervals in order to determine how it disappears naturally. In other words, we must investigate the degree of stability of the fixed set and how it disappears in the course of time.

Attention to this problem was first drawn by Fechner, and it was subsequently the subject of a special study by Stevens. The "motor set" which the latter describes may, in his opinion, persist for a fairly long period of time. However, Stevens made no special investigation of this problem, which was done for the first time in our laboratory [83].

A set was fixed in the subject over a period of 3 to 5 days (from 15 to 16 exposures). The critical experiments were carried out after intervals of different lengths (1 day, 2 to 3 days, 1 to 2 months). The experiments were carried out tachystoscopically, on optic illusions.

The results of these experiments are shown in Table XI. It is clear that the set, when fixed in these conditions, did not always disappear even 2 to 3 months after the first day of fixation. The figures show that this time, of course, modified the degree of fixation of the set, but the effect it had differed from case to case. In this respect, a considerable difference was often observed between our subjects. Whereas in some subjects the fixed set persisted for months, in others it disappeared comparatively early. In general, it can be said that the fixed set possesses a fairly high degree of stability, although on the other hand it must be admitted that the individual differences in this respect were very considerable.

The problem of the stability of the set is one awaiting investigation. It could have been examined more specifically in the above-

TABLE XI

Intervals	+	–	=
On the same day	54	12	34
After 1 day	75	5	20
After 2-3 days	75	5	20
After 2-3 months	62	12	26

mentioned investigation, carried out during the initial period of the study of the set, but at that time workers were concerned only with the problem of whether this phenomenon actually existed.

However, we must now consider how the set itself disappears, how the fixed set dies away under the influence of time. It must be assumed that the set, when exposed to this influence, gradually becomes weaker and ultimately disappears completely. Before the set becomes apparently extinguished, we must assume that it passes through a series of consecutive stages of gradual extinction.

2. Stages in the Process of Natural Disappearance of the Fixed Set

If we examine the state of the fixed set after a certain time interval, a definite picture emerges. We see the fixed set passes through definite stages of extinction, reaching, after a certain time, the state of total liquidation. We have essentially the same picture as with experimental extinction of the set. This provides the opportunity for examining the stages of natural suppression of the set.

We find that during the first days of the action of a fixed set, the dominant form of reaction is the contrast illusion. This is the same picture as when a fixed set is experimentally extinguished.

This stage of dominance of contrast illusions is followed by the stage of assimilative illusions. Of course, there is here no stage during which it could be said that assimilative illusions were present in a pure form. Both during the ordinary experimental extinction of the set and in this instance also, all that can be said is that this form of set appears and sometimes becomes predominant. All that need be said is that here we are actually dealing with a new phase in the process of disappearance of the set. In particular, when the set is extinguished naturally, this phase is represented in a comparatively purer form than during experimental extinction of the set. It is also found more frequently in natural conditions than in experimental conditions.

Finally, in the last stage, in addition to illusions we begin to see cases in which the equality of the critical objects is described, until eventually a stage is reached when no more illusions appear, and a stable evaluation of the critical objects is achieved. Both during the experimental extinction of the set and in the course of its natural extinction, it happens that in some subjects the set remains active for a longer time than in others. These are the cases in which the fixed set is not extinguished after what is regarded in experimental investigations as the maximal period (2 to 3 months in this case). It must be assumed that extinction of the set could occur after even longer periods.

Hence, the fixed set may be extinguished not only experimentally, but also naturally, and in both instances it happens in the same way; that is, the process of extinction occurs as a series of distinct phases following one another in a strictly definite order. In any case, this applies to a set fixed to quantitative relationships.

XI. THE ACTION OF CRITICAL EXPOSURES

1. The Fixing Action of Critical Experiments

We have seen that after a series of critical experiments, the fixed set is extinguished and replaced by a set more adequate to existing conditions. Admittedly, this does not always happen. As we know, a static, fixed set may frequently remain active. But normally, as a rule, only its dynamic form is encountered. This means that after a certain number of critical exposures (exposures of equal objects), the subject who is rid of his illusions begins to give correct answers. However, further experiments show that after some time—sooner in some cases, later in others—the illusions return and the subject's replies become inadequate. This conclusion is clear from our experiments on the stability of the set. The question accordingly arises: How can this be explained?

In order to solve this problem—one of great theoretical importance—special experiments were carried out designed to elucidate the situation arising as a result of our critical experiments. The purpose was to study how the repeated recognition of the equality of the objects in these experiments acts on the subject. Is a set toward equality fixed as a result of this repeated action of the critical objects, and in subsequent exposures are these objects identified as equal for the same reason?

In the experiments carried out to study this problem [5], the subjects witnessed the equality of the presented objects five times, and then in the critical series received figures differing only very slightly from each other in size: circles with a diameter of 20 to 21 mm, 20 to 22 mm, 20 to 23 mm, and 20 to 24 mm, and also squares measuring 15 to 16 mm, 15 to 17 mm, 15 to 18 mm, and 15 to 19 mm. The experiments were carried out in the following order: The subjects received in the fixing experiments a pair of circles (20 to 36 mm) 15 times. Next followed the critical experiments, a pair of equal circles (20 to 20 mm). After perceiving these circles as equal five times, the subjects were given unequal circles (20 to 21 mm) instead of the equal critical circles. If the circles continued to appear equal, they were again replaced, at first by circles of 20 to 22 mm, then 20 to 23 mm, and finally 20 to 24 mm.

What were the results of these experiments? From the exposure of a pair of critical circles 20 to 21 mm in diameter, the results shown in Table XII were obtained. It is clear that illusions arose in only 4 of the 46 subjects, while the remaining 42 gave perfectly adequate answers.

In the next series of experiments, the subjects were shown circles differing from each other in diameter by 2 mm. Still more revealing results were obtained in this instance; all 11 persons on whom the experiments were carried out (in this series, only those subjects who, in the preceding experiments, had had five successive illusions from the very beginning or after a short period of vacillation) described the critical circles as unequal.

In order to remove all doubt that in this instance the shape itself might have been a factor influencing the results, let us examine the results of the experiments with another shape, namely, the square. In these experiments, when the difference was 1 mm (15 to 16 mm) the results were precisely the same as those with

TABLE XII

	Illusions	Adequate
Absolute number	4	42
%	8.6	91.4

circles differing by the same amount in diameter. In fact, 3 persons had an illusion, while 43 evaluated the relationship between the figures quite correctly. So far as squares differing in size by 2 mm (15 to 17 mm) are concerned, the results obtained show that illusions were found only exceptionally (3 of 43 subjects), while a correct answer was the rule.

We do not give the results obtained in the other series of experiments on this problem (shaded circles instead of unshaded in the first series, unshaded squares instead of shaded in the preceding series); essentially, they substantiated the conclusions of the previous experiments and added nothing significant.

Hence, we may assume that the frequent repetition of reactions of equality to objects which actually are unequal in the critical experiments can by no means be taken to imply fixation of this equality.

But this conclusion can be valid only if we are convinced that the critical objects are perceived adequately, that is, as unequal, as a result of the absence of a set fixed on equality, and not because the inequality of the critical objects was excessively obvious and could not therefore be assimilated by a set fixed on equality.

It was essential to verify this hypothesis. Let us assume that we have a set fixed specially on equality, and let us present to a subject with such a set, as critical objects, the figures which we have been discussing (circles differing in radius by 1 or 2 mm). If the set is in fact unable to assimilate this difference, we shall obtain correct answers from the subject concerning the inequality of the figures presented to him; if not, then these figures will appear equal.

It is not difficult to verify this. However, it is unnecessary. We have already carried out experiments which will provide the answer to the question [43]. In these experiments, a set on the equality of geometrical figures (circles and squares) was fixed in a group of subjects, and they were then shown as critical object figures differing from each other in size by 1.5 and 1 mm (circles with a diameter of 22.5 and 24 mm and squares with sides measuring 21 and 22 mm in length). The results were in full agreement with the hypotheses mentioned above. The total number of subjects giving an illusion to at least one of the critical figures under the influence of the fixing experiment was 30, that is, 70.1% of the 42 subjects.

Consequently, it is conclusively established that in the presence of an appropriate set a difference in size between figures of 1 or 2 mm is of no importance; it does not prevent the manifestation of the assimilating effects of the fixed set.

This means that in the experiments described above, a difference of 1 or 2 mm in the size of the figures never went unnoticed; that is, these differences were never assimilated and there was no corresponding fixed set.

It may thus be regarded as well-established that in our usual experiments the repeated apperception of equal circles as equal never plays the role of the fixing presentations and never fixes a new and corresponding set. So long as equal figures are perceived as unequal, the whole of the set fixed in the preliminary experiments continues to act. When, however, the subject begins to perceive them repeatedly as equal, this is based, not on a set fixed on equality, but on a new set corresponding to the true situation.

Hence, there is no doubt that the critical exposures do not fix a new set. They merely accompany the manifestation of a set which is relevant to the current situation.

2. Temporary Extinction of the Set

As mentioned above, a short time after the end of the critical experiments, the repeated presentation of these experiments begins to produce the same customary illusions of the set. How can this be explained?

There is no doubt that as a result of critical exposures the previously fixed set is not finally abolished. In all probability, it withdraws in the face of a continuous series of critical exposures not fully corresponding to it, giving way to a more adequate set. When the set produced in the fixing experiments is stable enough, this takes place only temporarily, under the influence of the constant uninterrupted action of the critical exposures. Consequently, as soon as this period of continuous action of critical exposures is over, the strength of fixation again makes its presence felt, and revives the customary illusions of the set appropriate to it.

It must therefore be assumed that in the experiments on the stability of the set, we obtain results suggesting the continued survival of the fixed set. However, this survival is limited; after a certain time—in some cases sooner, in others later—the fixed set eventually dies away and never again opposes the development of new sets more adequate to the real situation.

3. The Problem of Asymmetry

It is therefore necessary to point out here one further fact. We know from ordinary observations and, in particular, from special experiments that man is essentially not constructed perfectly symmetrically. The best known example of human asymmetry is the functional inequality of our hands. A less obvious difference in this respect is found in the functioning of our other organs: legs, eyes, ears. In these cases, the functional inequality rests on a more or less obvious morphological difference between the organs.

Special investigations into the problem of asymmetry have revealed striking facts concerning its distribution. When in our experiments the subject receives two identical impressions (optic, haptic, or any other) for comparison with each other, in many instances the comparison is not made precisely or symmetrically, and one member of the relationship as a rule is overestimated in one way or another [91].

Consequently, we cannot be sure what determines the subject's remarks in each individual case, whether it is the evaluation of the objective situation or its subjective property—its asymmetry.

Besides the phenomena of asymmetry in the functioning of these organs, analogous phenomena have also been described in other instances where there is evidently no morphological basis for them. Consequently, the need arises for discussing the facts of "functional asymmetry." These facts require detailed study because phenomena of this type are widespread.

Special investigations, especially in the field of experimental psychophysical research, have shown us how rare is the adequate evaluation of the equality of the impressions which we receive from a wide range of different sensory sources. It may be taken as experimentally established that man generally perceives phenomena of inequality more easily and assesses them more correctly than phenomena of equality. This shows that man is more probably constructed in such a way as to perceive the environment asymmetrically than contrariwise, and that in general he is mentally inclined more toward phenomena of asymmetry than symmetry.

How can this be explained? To answer this question, we shall first try to determine whether it is possible to create artificially or experimentally in man a tendency toward the asymmetrical perception of impressions acting upon him.

We know that in our fixing experiments we were concerned in every instance with the experimentally stimulated asymmetry of our subjects. When, as a result of a series of fixing exposures, a corresponding set was fixed in the subject, thereafter for a definite period of time in critical experiments he began to exhibit stable asymmetry of perception: Of the two equal objects, one appeared larger than the other.

The impression obtained in this instance was precisely the same as that which we receive when we witness asymmetrical perceptions in persons who are found to be asymmetrical without any special measures. We are therefore justified in asking whether the phenomena of asymmetry in both cases may not rest on the same basis.

It is quite clear that neither in the case of our experimental asymmetry nor in the case of natural asymmetry is there in our subjects an organic defect which could serve as the basis for the phenomenon of asymmetry of perception. In none of these cases was the asymmetry organic in character. In experimental asymmetry, it rests on a set which was fixed as a result of the presentation of our fixing exposures. It is not impossible that in "natural" asymmetry we are dealing with a similar phenomenon. Admittedly, no special fixing exposures are received in such cases. This does not mean, however, that in the ordinary conditions of life a man may not find himself in a situation which acts on his set in the same fixing manner as took place in our experiments. Of course, in experiments we may act on the subject frequently and repeatedly for this purpose, although we know that this method is unnecessary for fixation of the set: Fixation may also arise as a result of a single presentation of a suitable situation. It must be assumed that in the life of each of us we may frequently encounter situations which, without any repetition, will fix the corresponding set. There is nothing, therefore, to prevent us from assuming that in the ordinary conditions of our life circumstances may arise which will at once fix the corresponding set.

We may accordingly conclude that each one of us carries within himself an innumerable multitude of sets fixed in the course of life which, when activated by a suitable condition, regulate the working of our mind in the corresponding direction.

It must also be noted that, as we have seen, as a result of the action of our critical exposures the fixed set may die away, allowing new sets, more adequate to the situation, to take over. The subject's experiences are determined now by the new set, and his replies are in line with it. This is what happens in our usual experiments. Briefly, after a few critical exposures, a set adequate to the particular situation takes control, and the one which was fixed in experimental conditions disappears completely at a certain moment.

What happens in the case of asymmetry, that is, in those cases in which we are dealing with "naturally" rather than experimentally fixed sets? How do the critical experiments act in this case? Do they have the same effect as in experimental conditions, or do they assume a different form here?

The only justification for stating the problem in this way is that the sets fixed in this case are of unconfirmed, and therefore unknown, origin. Despite this fact, however, they still remain ordinary fixed sets, and consequently they must share the fate of such sets in corresponding conditions.

This means that there are no grounds for assuming a different fate for naturally fixed sets than for experimentally fixed sets. If, as a result of the action of equal critical objects, a set fixed in experimental conditions is extinguished and a more relevant set takes over, then the same will also take place with the naturally fixed set; in these conditions, it also must be superseded by a set more adequate to the actual situation.

Hence, we see that in the critical experiments, nothing is left of the asymmetry which hitherto made itself felt so strongly; there is no difference in this case with whatever subject we are concerned—with the one who shows definite asymmetry or the one who appears to us to be perfectly symmetrical. On the whole, these facts suggest that in our experiments the phenomena of asymmetry do not play a role which calls for any special consideration.

XII. SETS ARISING ON THE BASIS OF THE QUALITY OF MATERIAL

It has been mentioned above that our ordinary experiments with sets are concerned with quantitative relationships and that aspects of quality are ignored. We must now ask ourselves whether these experiments must be regarded as being specific for quantitative relationships, and therefore unsuited for the examination of phenomena of other categories, in particular, the category of quality, or whether they may also be valid for qualitative phenomena.

1. Experiments on Sets Based on Equality

Before describing the results which we obtained in experiments on purely qualitative material, we must familiarize ourselves with the results of investigations in which the problem was formulated rather differently. The question being asked is: What happens if a subject is given a series of stimuli in order to produce a fixed set to equality rather than to difference and then in critical experiments is shown a pair of unequal objects and asked to compare them ? We have here, of course, all the conditions regarded as sufficient for obtaining fixation of the set. However, it is quite clear that this cannot be a set based on a relationship of "larger" or "smaller." Consequently, in this situation no illusions of contrast may be obtained.

Therefore, we are here dealing with experiments in conditions almost completely identical to those in our usual experiments, but without the possibility of contrast illusions occurring. What are the results obtained in these experiments [43] ?

Before answering this question, we must draw attention to the special position occupied among other relationships by the equality relationship. The phenomena evolving around us obviously differ from each other in some respect; no absolutely identical phenomena can exist. Equality or identity may be determined only after we have observed objective phenomena for a specific purpose—in order to relate a particular phenomenon to the world of phenomena in general. In fact, equality can be determined only in the form of identity, that is, only in relation to itself. Accordingly, it is clear that objects can only be equal if they belong to the world of artificial phenomena, created by human hands, and not to the world of natural objects.

If, however, we accept that this is so, it becomes clear that the observation of relationships of equality is much more difficult than the observation of relationships of inequality. It is not surprising, therefore, that the repetition of experiments in order to fix a set based on equality should meet with difficulties which are not encountered in the experiments with sets based on "larger" or "smaller." Special measures must therefore be taken in these experiments in order to enable our subject to perceive the objects presented to him repeatedly as equal. It will suffice for this purpose to draw the subject's attention to the "equality" of the fixing objects.

Without discussing the other measures which must be taken to facilitate the fixation of a set based on equality, I must dwell for a while on the problem of critical stimuli. As shown above, critical stimuli must always be equal objects. In our experiments, it will be remembered, the problem arose of the degree of inequality between objects permissible here.

It was easy to show that the inequality must be only very slightly above the threshold level, since if the difference was too great, it could not be assimilated. As critical objects circles differing by 1.5 mm in diameter and squares whose sides differed in length by 1 mm could be used. Possibly, however, this difference could be inadequate for some of the subjects.

Accordingly, the experiments were usually conducted as follows: At the beginning the subjects were shown the figures of the critical experiments, and if they could not identify them as obviously different, they were replaced by others differing more from each other.

The first result of these experiments to be noted is that, because of the absence of conditions favoring the development of illusions of contrast, no such illusions were observed. Conversely, assimilative illusions were predominant, for they occurred in 70.1% of subjects in whom a fixed set had been formed; unequal circles or squares appeared as a rule to be always equal.

Consequently, it is clear that in these conditions, that is, essentially in the usual conditions of development of our illusions of the set, new illusions may appear which may be described as illusions of a set based on inequality. This is the first and most important result obtained from these experiments, by which they differ from the usual experiments with sets.

What happens to the other features observed in similar cases? In the first place, it is found that the excitability of the set in this instance can be investigated in the ordinary way, just as in our quantitative experiments. However, as might have been expected, the results obtained are somewhat unusual. In fact, the excitability of a fixed set based on equality is much lower than in cases with a set fixed on other quantitative relationships. When working with sets of this type it is important always to bear in mind that a set based on equality is more difficult to fix and is fixed later than one based on inequality. In concrete terms, fixation is at best achieved in 12 to 15 fixing exposures. In other cases the number of fixing exposures may reach 25 to 30.

Hence, we may repeat that a set to a relationship of equality is appreciably more difficult to fix than the usual quantitative set.

It is interesting to examine the course of extinction of a set based on equality. This is particularly interesting because the phenomenon of illusions of contrast is absent here, and, as we have learned, this phenomenon plays a particularly important part during the succession of stages of extinction of the set.

If, however, cases of illusions of contrast are completely excluded, only two possibilities remain: assimilative illusions and adequate responses. In our experiments on sets based on equality we obtain both these possibilities; most frequently a series of responses is observed in which the subjects give either a continuous series of assimilative illusions or, on the other hand, after giving a few such illusions a sharp change is made to adequate responses.

This, however, is not the only type of reaction given by the subjects in these experiments. Cases of a different type may be found: The subject gives, not a continuous series of illusions, but illusions interspersed with correct responses. However, this interchange of reactions stops after a short time and gives way to a continuous series of correct evaluations of the critical figures. In this case, therefore, we are dealing with phenomena reminiscent of the third stage in the usual process of extinction of fixed sets.

Hence, in experiments on inequality we do not find the wealth of phases characteristic of the course of extinction of the fixed set based on "bigger" and "smaller." Considering the nature of these experiments, it could not be otherwise. Nevertheless, we have no grounds for assuming that a fixed set based on equality is extinguished immediately and not gradually; the presence of a third phase, that is, a phase of assessment as unequal, in any case is not in doubt. It must be noted, however, that in these experiments the incidence of static sets, that is, the number of persistent illusions, is comparatively high (20% of the total).

The problem of the degree of stability of fixed sets based on equality merits particular attention. The facts relating to this problem are as follows:

A. After a pause of 15 to 20 min, a fixed set remains active in only 38% of subjects (5 of 13). This quite conclusively demonstrates the very low stability of our fixed set based on equality. If it is borne in mind that in 3 of these 5 persons the set was so weak that it disappeared after 1 to 4 exposures, there can be no doubt about the conclusion of the low stability of sets based on equality.

B. So far as the possibility that such a fixed set may last for a longer time, for example, 24 hours, the results of these experiments do not confirm it. In any case, no conclusive results were obtained to support this possibility.

C. The results of our experimental investigations on the set have shown conclusively, as mentioned above, that a set fixed on particular material (let us say, on circles) may be transferred without difficulty to another material (let us say, for example, to squares) so that the set becomes generalized.

We know that in our usual experiments generalization of the set takes place usually to such a degree that, if it is not taken into consideration, the true importance of these experiments cannot be realized. In order to show that in experiments on equality we are dealing essentially with ordinary fixed sets, we must dwell longer on experiments concerned with the possibility of generalization of these sets.

Experiments were carried out on subjects in whom a set based on equality was fixed precisely and definitely. To verify that generalization of the set established in this subject took place, only circles and squares were used. Tests were carried out to discover whether the set based on equality in the case of circles also extended to squares.

These experiments showed that the phenomenon of generalization also occurred in these experiments. It was found that a set based on equality of circles was generalized to squares, and vice versa. The fact discovered in the experiments with sets based on relationships of "larger" and "smaller" also applied in this instance.

Consequently, an examination of all these facts reveals clearly that in experiments on equality basically the same results are obtained as in our ordinary fixing experiments.

Hence, it may be concluded that these experiments are precisely the same fixing experiment, but carried out with different material. They are of great interest to us, especially in the respect that they lead us directly to the question of the possible extension of the results obtained in fixing experiments on quantitative relationships between "larger" and "smaller" to the field of relationships of equality. If we could show that this was so, that the concept of the fixed set was equally applicable here, the results of our experiments could be used not only to define a set based on quantitative relationships, but equally well to define a set based on qualitative relationships, for it is an undoubted fact that equality belongs to some extent to the category of quality. Let us now go on to consider this problem [109].

2. Experiments with Fixed Sets Based on Qualitative Differences

In our laboratories we have made several attempts to investigate sets based on qualitatively different relationships [109]. Here we shall describe only one of these investigations directly concerned with the problem on which we are engaged. We have already mentioned this investigation above, and have described in general terms the method used. It was then stated that the method was designed for the investigation of purely qualitative relationships and was perfectly suitable for defining them. We can now examine more fully the results obtained in these investigations.

The subject is given with a tachystoscope a series of words (30 in number) written in Latin characters with five letters in each: for example, ridal, daluf, tifal, and so on. He is then given a series of Russian words (35 or more) each containing five letters. These were written in a neutral handwriting, and could also be read as if they were Latin words: for example, почва, топор, рупор, and so on. The first series of words in Latin handwriting was used as fixing objects and the second series as critical objects. The problems of the excitability and stability of the set and particularly the phases of the set were studied. The results of these experiments are given below. The first feature to attract attention was that in this case the set based on reading Latin words was quite definitely fixed; having read a series of words, the subject persisted in reading them as Latin. The subsequent Russian words played the role of critical objects, and the subject read them in accordance with the previously fixed set as Latin words. For example, instead of the perfectly familiar Russian word топор, the subject read "монон," and instead of порча he said "нонра" and so on.

It was next found that the set was fixed in all the subjects; they all conformed to the set based on reading in Latin and accordingly could not guess that the words порча, топор, and so on, were Russian and not Latin. In the course of time, however, they realized that they were looking at Russian words. Of course, not all subjects behave in the same way; some change to reading in Russian sooner, others later; some do so at once, others gradually, and so on.

The interesting discovery was made that in these experiments the fixed set disappears, passing through several distinct phases as it does so.

A. The first feature to attract attention was that the subject did not begin with illusions of contrast, as in our usual experiments. Their place was taken by the usual assimilative illusion; the subject read the Russian words as if they had been Latin. We have already mentioned this above, where we noted it as a specific feature of qualitative experiments with sets. In fact, this is the only difference between these experiments and the usual experiments with sets. It must be concluded that our views regarding illusions of contrast, which we have already discussed above, correspond sufficiently closely to the true state of affairs. The phenomenon of contrast is one which is characteristic only of the category of intensity—the qualitative sphere of reality is not concerned with contrast.

B. The second stage of regressive development of the set in the reading experiments may be described as follows: At first, the subject reads with mixed assimilation [109] (for example, he reads "топор" as "мопор" or " моноп "; that is, some letters are read as Latin letters and some as Russian). However, such "mixed assimilation" is always less frequent than reading in Latin. Hence, the characteristic feature of this second stage is reading with "mixed assimilation." The number of subjects in the group reading with mixed assimilation may reach 60% of the total taking part in the experiment.

C. Since a few cases of mixed assimilation are followed by cases of reading sometimes in Russian and sometimes in Latin, but more rarely in Russian (that is, correctly), then in these cases we may describe a third stage of the regressive development of the fixed set. Reading in this manner is found comparatively more often than is the preceding second stage of regressive development of the set. Of the total number of subjects, 73.3% passed through this stage, whereas in the second stage we found at most only 60% of subjects.

The next stages are characterized as follows: stage 4, reading mainly in Russian; stage 5, reading Russian words, as Latin, but with rapid correction and correct pronunciation (30% of subjects); and finally stage 6, characterized by generally correct reading of all Russian words, but with preliminary apperception of some of these words as Latin, and rapid suppression of these involuntary apperceptions by correct reading in Russian (40% of subjects).

D. If we examine more closely these stages of regressive development of the set, it is easy to see that here we are dealing essentially, or at any rate from the practical point of view, not with six but with only three stages of regressive development of the fixed set. The fact is that all four stages (3, 4, 5, and 6) following the second stage can be combined into a single third stage of development of the set. The characteristic feature of this stage would then be predominance of reading in Russian over reading in Latin. This would then be followed eventually by the complete extinction of the fixed set and of the incorrect reading of the presented series of words. If we were to restrict ourselves to the differentiation of only these main stages of regressive development of this particular set, we would find a fundamental analogy between the two types of sets—between qualitative and quantitative sets. We would then say that basically the mechanism of the set is the same whatever it is concerned with—regardless of whether quantitative or qualitative material.

This situation holds good if we ask ourselves whether in these qualitative experiments we can find the special features characteristic of sets based on quantitative relationships.

But can we, in fact, speak of indices of stability of the set in these experiments? We may remember that by stability of the set we mean that property which results in its being able to withstand the action of conflicting stimuli and remain undisturbed. It is clear that this feature of the set must show itself, above all, in the duration of the first stage of regressive development, expressing its assimilative powers. Consequently, to test the degree of stability of a set and to measure it, we must establish the number of critical exposures necessary in each individual case to produce final suppression of the set. The results thus obtained enable us to judge the stability of the set as follows: Reading, for example, 5 to 7 words under the assimilating influence of the set points to a weak degree of stability of the set (26.9% of the total number of subjects), 8 to 11 words denotes an average degree (55.2%), and finally 12 words or more indicates a high degree of stability of the set (66.7%).

It is interesting, however, to examine what happens with a number of repetitions of the fixing exposures recognized as absolutely adequate for producing a set firmly fixed on qualitative differences.

As we have seen above, a set based on the relationship between the volumes of certain articles is more stable the greater the number of preliminary exposures used in its fixation. In much the same way it must be assumed that the stability or strength of a set based on qualitative determinations is measured by the number of words assimilated by the action of a particular number of fixing units; in fact, the experiments showed that after 5 fixing words their assimilating influence extended only to 1 or 2 words; after 15 such words, 4 or 5 words were assimilated; and after 30, 5 to 10 words.

Without discussing the other results of these experiments, the general conclusion can be drawn that the stability of a fixed set based on apperception of Latin words is directly dependent on the number of fixing exposures used in each individual case. Consequently, the stability of a fixed set is undoubtedly measurable also in qualitative experiments.

Let us now turn briefly to the question of the excitability of qualitative sets. It has been found that in suitable conditions its magnitude can be measured. First, its value is not constant—it varies with the individual makeup of the subject. Whereas with some subjects one fixing Latin word was enough to ensure that the subsequent Russian words were completely assimilated, with others the number of fixing words had to be greater than one, and it differed from one person to another. Consequently, the excitability of qualitative sets is a value which varies from one individual to another.

Second, compared with indices of excitability of a set based on quantitative relationships, excitability to qualitative data is considerably higher. While one single Latin word was sufficient to fix the corresponding set (in 80% of all cases), in quantitative experiments 4 repetitions of optical exposures were required to obtain fixation for the first time, and, moreover, within very wide limits (29.5% of subjects).

Finally, we might have expected that in these experiments we could examine the problem of the stability of the set. It was discovered that:

A. The set is maintained after an interval of one day in 60% of cases, whereas on the same day it is exhibited in all cases without exception. After longer intervals—one month, let us say—the coefficient of preservation of the set falls to 25% of all cases. Hence, with lengthening of the interval between the fixing and critical experiments, the percentage of cases of activity of the set falls considerably, but nevertheless it persists to some degree for a long time.

B. As the length of the interval between the fixing and critical experiments increases, the set, although still preserved, becomes increasingly less plastic. For example, after one day it still passes through all three stages (1–4%, 2–10%, and 4–10%), whereas after an interval of one month it loses all its plasticity, which remains only in the first stage of its manifestation.

C. In connection with the question of the stability of the set, one further fact may be mentioned: After an interval of 24 hours, one of the subjects read 8 Russian words in succession in Latin, and the other 3 subjects read 4 or 5 words in this manner, after which their reading was adequate and correct. After an interval of one month the indices were lower still; one subject read the first 3 Russian words as Latin, and the other two subjects the first 2 words.

The results obtained may be expressed in general terms as follows: A set fixed on reading in Latin continues to exist for some time, but to exist so that as the time interval increases, its manifestation becomes steadily weaker, and this is shown by a decrease in both its total and its phased activity [109].

3. Special Features of a Set Fixed on Qualitative Differences

What special features are observed in the process of extinction of a set fixed on qualitative material?

First, it must be noted that we never find the first stage of extinction of the set—we do not find the illusions of contrast observed in the initial stages of extinction of a set fixed on quantitative relationships. Instead, we begin straightaway with assimilative illusions—with the effect of the direct action of the fixed set on the subject's perception.

This fact emphasizes once again that the presence of contrast is specific only to the perception of quantitative relationships, and that qualitative properties, on the contrary, are characterized by the complexity of their interrelationships. Consequently, a phenomenon resulting from the specific properties of quantitative relationships cannot be regarded as a specific feature of the set itself; it grows out of the intrinsic properties of the material, but it is not part of the nature of the set itself.

A set based on qualitative relationships does not include a stage of illusions of contrast, since it is a stage resulting from some specific aspect of the material of quantitative relationships and not from the special features of the set itself.

The process of extinction of the set is essentially a much simpler process than might have been expected judging from the observations made on the stages of extinction of sets based on quantitative relationships.

If the stage of illusions of contrast is excluded, the process of extinction of the fixed set may be represented as follows: (1) Initially we may have illusions of assimilation where Russian words are read as Latin. (2) This is followed by a stage of mixed assimilative illusions and adequate perceptions where, for example, in the presence of a set fixed on reading a Latin text, the subject may read the word чурек as чупек, that is, as a mixture of Russian and Latin (in this case the third letter is read as Latin and the others as Russian). (3) Next follows essentially the last stage, that of reading the presented words sometimes as Russian, sometimes as Latin.

The process of extinction of a set fixed on quantitative relationships is undoubtedly much more complex than the same process with a set fixed on qualitative material. Nevertheless, in the process of extinction of a fixed set in this last case we find a stage which is not found at all during the extinction of quantitative sets. This is the second stage, that is, the stage of "mixed assimilation," in which the subject reads the same words sometimes as Russian and sometimes as Latin.

The presence of this stage may also be detected by another series of experiments with sets based on qualitative relationships. For example, in the experiments carried out by my colleague N. L. Eliava, who fixed a set on a picture with a definite meaning, it was found that in the critical experiments the subjects perceived a new picture presented to them on the basis of the same mixed assimilation as in the experiments on reading in Latin; that is, they saw a picture which combined the signs not only of the critical picture but also of the fixing picture.

To summarize, in experiments with sets based on qualitative differences, a special stage of the process of extinction of the fixed set appears, characterized by combined assimilation of some of the signs of both the fixing and the critical objects.

We find nothing like this in experiments with sets based on quantitative relationships. The situation there is completely different; the stage of illusion of contrast is followed by a stage of assimilative or mixed illusions with perceptions of equality, and finally, a stage of completely adequate responses appears. Here, in each individual case, one of two things happens—either a relationship of equality or a relationship of inequality ("larger" or "smaller"). Other signs in this case may or may not be present, for since quantitative relationships are mutually exclusive, it is impossible that the members of a relationship could be equal and unequal at the same time.

It is another matter with sets based on qualitative properties. We saw above that in one stage of the regressive development of the fixed set a specific form of illusion appears, consisting of the apparently simultaneous manifestation of the activity of two states of the set—a state created in the fixing experiments and a state adequate to the perception of the critical objects. For example, when presented with the Russian word чурек as critical stimulus, the subject reads it as чупек , perceiving the Russian letter "p" (=r) as the Latin letter "p". The same phenomenon is observed quite frequently in all other experiments with sets based on qualitative relationships. The subject, for example, perceives a picture of critical objects as a new image including elements of both the fixing and the critical pictures.

How can this new image apparently represent the product of two separate but simultaneously acting sets? If we remember that any set is an integral state of the personality, then it seems impossible that there could be any such product, representing as it were a mixture of various elements of two independent sets.

But how can this phenomenon be understood? In the experiments with reading a text, we may draw attention to one distinctive feature which was apparent only in these experiments but which nevertheless is of general importance. I refer to the following: When, after a series of Latin fixing presentations, the subject was asked to read the Russian word чурек, and he read it as чупек, this means that this word was not perceived at all as a Russian word, despite the fact that all the letters except one, or at least the first two, were read by the subject as Russian letters. The combination of letters before the subject's eyes (ч-у-р-е-к) did not represent a true word to him because this word in the first place had the value of this particular group of sounds; when this value, as in this case, is zero, or when I cannot see it, then the word breaks up into a simple group of sounds, completely disconnected. Each separate letter in this case becomes an independent unit which can be read according to any adequate alphabet so that nothing is disturbed except, perhaps, the set of reading in accordance with a definite alphabet. This set, however, if it does not sustain the meaning of what is perceived in each individual case, easily dies away and is replaced by another set, fixed on a different basis.

In brief, when I read a combination of letters, irrespective of the meaning which they express, there is no basis for reading them in accordance with any particular language. It easily happens, therefore, that in these cases a group of letters disintegrates into individual units, which some subjects may perceive as letters of one alphabet and other subjects as those of another alphabet. We see here another manifestation of the reduplication of the set which we mentioned above.

But what happens in other cases, in the experiments with pictures? As we have seen, it sometimes happens that subjects, after a series of fixing experiments with a certain picture, begin to perceive a new picture presented to them in critical experiments as a complex image incorporating elements of both the fixing and the critical pictures. In other words, we are confronted with exactly the same phenomena as in the experiments on reading in Latin. The only difference is that whereas in the first case we were dealing only with a combination of letters, irrespective of the meaning which they possibly contained, in this case we are dealing with pictures which are pictures anyhow, and which are therefore always perceived as meaningful entities. Hence, in this case we are dealing of necessity with pictures or illustrations of something, and not with an empty, meaningless combination of lines or colors. In these experiments, therefore, we do not obtain an exact repetition of the results which we saw in the experiments on reading.

Does this mean, however, that in these experiments we must recognize the presence of two completely independent, unconnected sets at the same time in the subject? If we analyze cases of this type, we see that the answer to this question must be in the negative. When in critical experiments the subject sees a picture which apparently combines the features of both the fixing and the critical objects, this certainly does not mean that in this case we are dealing in fact with a combined picture. On the contrary, the picture perceived is a single, completely whole image, which is certainly not a combined representation of the pictures presented in these experiments. A mere glance at it is enough to see that it is a completely independent, integral picture in which a careful analysis reveals only elements taken from the pattern of the fixing picture.

However, if this is so it proves that in the critical experiments we are not dealing with the appearance and the combined activity of two sets, but with the formation of a specific set, lying at the basis of perception of the form of the critical objects.

Hence, the course of the set fixed on qualitative material so closely resembles that of the ordinary quantitative set that it does not seem necessary to study them separately. For the investigation of sets in general it would seem sufficient to use only one of these methods. At the present time, we prefer the method with sets fixed on quantitative relationships, because they are comparatively more highly developed and in most instances we shall continue to use them.

XIII. THE DIFFERENTIAL PSYCHOLOGY OF THE SET

A general psychological analysis of the phenomena of the set shows that it is an essential factor largely determining the structure of human behavior. Besides this, however, evidence has been obtained indicating the differential psychological importance of the study of problems concerning the set. We have seen that the phenomena of the set do not always and everywhere follow the same course, and that in some cases it may change its normal course of activity and become abnormal. This makes it necessary to consider the problem of the set in more detail from differential psychological points of view. We should not be surprised to find that the set is a factor in human psychology endowed with considerable differential importance.

1. Differentiation of the Set

In the first place, we must consider the question of differentiation of the set, lying at the basis of certain manifestations of human behavior. We know that usually in the course of the experience of a particular individual, a certain number of repeated presentations of a given stimulus is necessary before the appropriate set is defined and differentiated. The question therefore naturally arises: What is the importance of the individual factor in this case? It would not be surprising to find that the course of differentiation of the set is not absolutely identical in all cases or in all individuals. If we find that this is so, the investigation of the process of differentiation of the set in each particular case would have to be recognized as an essentially important problem in differential psychology.

If we assume that the set plays the role in the psychology of behavior which we have ascribed to it, it is clear that the behavior of each individual is largely dependent on the course of differentiation of his sets, on the speed with which they are formed, and on the degree to which they are defined. Confused behavior, indecisiveness, and vagueness are the natural result of the low level of differentiation of the set lying at the basis of this behavior. On the other hand, dilatoriness and inability to make decisions in essential actions must be regarded as the natural result of this specific quality of the process of differentiation of the set.

Several observations have shown conclusively that people differ considerably in behavior. It should therefore be realized that the processes of differentiation of their sets will also differ significantly. Clearly, therefore, the detection and definition of the distinctive rate and path of differentiation of the set in each individual case is one of the more important differential psychological problems awaiting solution in the psychology of set. Despite this, no experimental investigations of this problem have yet been carried out.

2. Excitability of the Fixed Set

We have drawn attention above to the true meaning of this concept. We know that before a set can be fixed, a definite number of fixing experiments must be carried out. We have not yet mentioned, however, that this number must not be regarded as a fixed value, equally applicable to the set of every individual. On the contrary, our numerous experiments have shown that this number is dependent on the differential psychological category. There are some persons in whom the set is fixed from the very beginning—the set is fixed firmly enough after the first presentation, whereas on the other hand we may meet other persons who give the impression that their sets are almost impossible to fix. Admittedly, these two extremes are met comparatively rarely, but nevertheless they are borderline cases and their presence has been proved beyond doubt. Of course, a sufficiently large number of fixing exposures will ultimately fix the set even in this latter case. Between these extremes there are intermediate states varying from low to very high values of the number of fixing exposures required.

When considering the data concerning the excitability of the set in individuals, it must be borne in mind from the outset that these facts must be first selected from a particular point of view. It is essential to know when and after how many fixing experiments definite and incontrovertible traces of fixation may be recognized.

As mentioned above, many experiments concerned with sets have shown us that in this respect individuals differ considerably from each other; in some persons fixation of the set is observed comparatively early, but in others the first signs of fixation do not appear until very late.

During the study of the set it is sometimes extremely important to know when the set first begins to show signs of fixation. Here also it is necessary to study the excitability of the set from the first moments of its appearance.

However, this is by no means the extent of the problem of excitability. We may have to consider the optimal degree of excitability, that is, the relative degree of excitation which is most suitable for the set of a particular individual. As might be expected, the indices of two forms of excitability do not coincide; in some persons the threshold of minimal and optimal excitability are far removed, whereas in other persons these thresholds may be close together.

A complete definition of the excitability of a fixed set in a particular person requires both these thresholds to be established. Depending on the difference in their values we may frequently find specific distinguishing features in the behavior of subjects who otherwise resemble each other very considerably. The thresholds of excitability are very easily determined. They are measured by the number of fixing exposures required for (1) the initial degrees of fixation of the set (indices of the lower threshold) and (2) the optimal degrees of fixation (indices of the optimal threshold).

3. Excitability of the Fixed Set in Children

Besides the individual factor, the age factor is also concerned here; we know from special investigations of the fixed set in children that its excitability is one of the main features distinguishing this age period, in particular the preschool period [88]. It has now been firmly established that a single fixing exposure may be sufficient to fix a set in a child of this age group. In 80% of preschool children investigated, a fixed set appeared after a single exposure. Assimilative illusions were observed in 60% and illusions of contrast in 20% of the children studied.

Hence, it is clear that the excitability of the initial degrees of fixation of the set in the preschool age is very high, but at the same time it can also be seen that in the initial levels of excitability we find low indices of fixation, characterized by the predominance of assimilative illusions.

With an increase in the number of fixing exposures to 4, the state of affairs becomes very different; now the predominant form of reaction becomes the illusion of contrast, and the number of assimilative illusions falls to 25%. With a further increase in the number of fixing experiments (15 exposures), the number of illusions of contrast shows another significant increase (74 to 79%), but not to such an extent that it should be regarded as the optimal number.

However, at this stage we encounter a factor which must be considered further. This is the stability of the fixed set, which gives significantly high indices after a further increase in the number of fixing experiments. The number of illusions of contrast now rises to 67%, compared to barely 40% after 4 exposures. At the same time, the number of assimilative illusions falls considerably (after 2 exposures 30%, after 4 to 8 exposures 10 to 12%, and after 15 exposures 6%). These results suggest that the optimal number of fixing exposures in preschool age should be regarded as 15 rather than 4.

It can therefore be concluded that the excitability of the set in children of preschool age is comparatively high; its lower threshold is not greater than 1, while its optimal threshold although not 4, is in any case not greater than 15.

Turning now to school age, we find that the coefficient of excitability of the set begins to rise higher still. However, we can evidently assume that this coefficient does not move appreciably away from the indices of the preschool age until the age of 11 years. This time interval in the life of the child—namely, preschool age and early school age—must clearly be regarded as the period of the greatest excitability of the set.

This period is followed by the middle school period—the ages of 12, 13, 14, and, in some cases, 15 years—characterized by a definite fall in the values of the indices of excitability.

After this period, at the ages of 15 to 17 years, the indices of excitability show a definite increase. Some doubt may perhaps be felt regarding the results for children aged 17 years, which fell significantly, according to reported investigations. However, in view of the very small number of children studied in this age period (only 10, compared to between 58 and 214 in other age groups), these indices had best be disregarded, and their values equated with those for adjacent age groups. In this case, a more definite picture of the development of the excitability of the fixed set in schoolchildren is observed, starting from the age of 15 years [88].

We find that the excitability of the set is very high in the preschool period, somewhat lower until the age of 11 years, then (12 to 14 years) falls sharply, to rise again between 15 and 17 years.

In psychopathological cases a distinctive picture of the excitability of the set is seen. There is reason to suppose, as we shall see below, that the excitability of the set in some pathological conditions may vary; in some cases, its indices may rise sharply, while in others they may fall just as sharply. As examples we may mention, on the one hand, certain types of schizophrenia in which the excitability of the set is very high and, on the other hand, types of psychasthenia in which the coefficient of excitability falls sharply. However, these phenomena will be discussed more fully below, in the chapter on psychopathological cases.

4. Stability of the Set

Our experiments also revealed that the next distinguishing feature of the set was the stability of its fixation. A wide range in degree of stability of the fixed set may be observed in different persons and in different situations.

In the first place, however, we must discuss what we mean by this property of the set. What exactly is its stability? It may be assumed that it is synonymous with the ease of formation of the set, and that persons in whom the set is easily fixed may be described as people with a stable set. But this is not necessarily so. On the contrary, it sometimes happens that a set fixed as a result of a large number of fixing exposures is much weaker than a set established after a comparatively shorter series of fixing experiments. The converse may also take place.

In brief, it must be concluded that the stability of the set and the ease of its fixation are completely independent phenomena. Whatever the true state of affairs, the problem which we are considering requires special study.

We may therefore assume that people differ from each other not only in the degree of excitability of the fixed set, but also in its stability. The question arises: How can the level of stability of the fixed set be determined experimentally?

As an index of the stability of the fixed set we may perhaps take the length of the path which must be followed by the subject before he can reach a state of complete extinction of a fixed set. This path may be measured in two ways: (1) After a series of fixing experiments we may present critical objects to the subject for a long time and then measure how long it takes him to identify them. The length of time required for this process is an index of the stability of the fixed set which we wish to measure. (2) The second method is based on the following argument: As the index of the duration of exposure of the critical objects we may take the number of repetitions before the subject clearly sees that they are equal. The results obtained by the second method are the same as those at the beginning of the experiment; as at first, the subject gives a series of incorrect answers, but then gradually becomes increasingly successful in giving the correct evaluation of the critical objects presented to him.

Hence, it may be concluded that the stability of the set may be measured both by the duration of the critical exposures and by the number of repeated and transient exposures of the critical objects.

We may thus see from a series of investigations of the fixed set in persons differing from each other in a number of signs that the stability of the set must be regarded as an index of definite differential psychological importance. However, no special investigation of this and similar problems has yet been carried out.

5. Dynamic and Static Sets

When a fixed set is already present, then regardless of how it was fixed, we have to consider its regressive development and the process of its extinction. This problem must be studied because the differential psychological nature of this phenomenon is clearly apparent during the study of the general psychological question of extinction of the fixed set. We have seen that the process of extinction of a fixed set possesses several common paths of development, but the individual psychological factor undoubtedly plays an important role.

What, then, are the differential psychological aspects of this problem? We pointed out above that there are two possible ways for the subject to solve the problem facing him in a particular situation. He may either suppress his set or he may be unable to do so. This factor alone is sufficient to show that we are essentially dealing not with a general psychological problem, but simply with a differential psychological problem. These two possibilities of reaction are mutually exclusive, which means that they cannot exist simultaneously in the same person.

We saw above that two types of persons can be distinguished according to this point of view. Persons who, as a result of passing through a series of stages, ultimately reach the stage of recognition of the equality of the critical figures we describe as subjects with a "dynamic" set. In this group we include all subjects who in our experiments usually described the equality of the critical objects and who, freed from the influence of the previously fixed set, began to solve the problem correctly.

Frequently, however, persons of the second type are encountered. These persons are unable to rid themselves of the influence of the fixed set which dominates them at the particular moment. Time evidently cannot weaken and ultimately eradicate a previously fixed set. We have seen above that in such cases we are dealing with persons with a "static" set.

In contrast to the dynamic set, the static set is not a form found among normal persons. Its distinguishing feature is that the subject for a long period of time remains under the influence of the same fixed set—a set which not only is inadequate itself, but which does not give the opportunity of appearing so. Persons with a static form of fixed set cannot be regarded as fully adapted subjects. They are quite definitely abnormal. For this reason it is not surprising that the static form of set is most frequently found in psychopathological cases. We shall see below how high the proportion of persons with this form of set is among the group of abnormal subjects whom we studied.

Nevertheless, it should not be concluded that a static set is a specific sign characteristic only of frankly abnormal subjects. This is clear from the extensive facts available for our analysis. These facts show that there are individual groups of people specifically characterized by the static nature of their sets, or who, among other features, may also carry this trait. Below, when we analyze the main typological groups, we shall discuss this problem specially. We shall see then that persons, for example, with a coarse, static set are usually a clearly defined type of person, not at all infrequently encountered.

Hence, the dynamic and static nature of the set are signs which must be taken into consideration in the differential psychological description of human subjects.

6. Plasticity and Coarseness of the Set

When we described the process of extinction of the fixed set above, we mentioned these aspects of it. We found then that the process of extinction of the set takes place in a definite order and that, in particular, its plastic and coarse or inert form must be distinguished. We must now emphasize that this feature is also important from the typological point of view, and during the study of individual persons these aspects cannot be avoided.

But what exactly are they? What do we mean, what aspects of the life of the set do we imply, when we discuss its plasticity and its coarseness or how else could we describe the property of its inertness? When we discussed the general psychological problems of the set above, we mentioned this question. We then discussed in adequate detail the differentiation between these forms. At this stage it is essential to emphasize which factor in the activities of the set they concern.

Whereas the dynamic or static nature of the set concerns its ultimate fate, namely, whether in the existing conditions it will be suppressed or whether this is impossible, in the present case, when determining the plasticity or coarseness of our sets we mean something completely different: Here it is its fate in the process of extinction, the changes which it undergoes in this process regardless of how it ends, whether it is extinguished or not. If a fixed set begins to yield under the influence of a series of critical experiments—to change, to become weaker, regardless of what eventually happens to it—we may describe the fixed set as plastic. If the process of the critical experiments has no effect on the character of the set and it persists until the end, evidently unchanged, in these cases we regard the set as coarse or inert.

Our experiments showed that these aspects of the set also have a well-defined differential psychological character. Such individual psychological value as they may possess will be discussed below. At this stage we must note that these features of the set, like its dynamic and static qualities mentioned above, are factors which vary depending on individual and (perhaps or) other conditions (age, sex, and so on).

In particular, with respect to the age changes in the development of the fixed set we have evidence which definitely confirms both their presence and the distinctive features of their progress [88]. Admittedly, they still need some amplification, but even in their present form they can still be useful in this context. We mentioned above that the optimal number of fixing experiments in children may be taken to be 15 exposures. I therefore consider that the most characteristic feature of children is the indices which they give as a result of fixation of the set under the influence of precisely this number of exposures. If we examine the available evidence concerning different age groups, we find that the main forms of set which we are discussing are distributed as follows: At preschool age, the dominant form is the static fixed set; in the early school period it is still the static set, but in a plastic form, and finally in the middle school period, a coarse dynamic set. Admittedly, these findings cannot be regarded as final, but at least they give us an approximate picture of the distribution of the forms of fixed set among different age groups.

7. Irradiation and Generalization of the Set

We have already encountered the problem of irradiation of the set. Now, however, we shall discuss this question only from the theoretical point of view, as a general psychological phenomenon. At this point we must state that this problem also has a differential psychological aspect.

Admittedly, the set is a psychological fact which has as one of its features, perhaps a specially important feature, the fact that it irradiates throughout the organism as a whole. On the other hand, however, we find evidence which shows that the degree of irradiation of the set cannot always be determined, or that in some cases it is wide, while in other cases it spreads only over a comparatively localized area. Since this is so, it shows conclusively that the problem of irradiation of the set may be included among the differential psychological problems.

When the problem of irradiation of the set is investigated from the general psychological point of view, we cannot, of course, entirely avoid this differential psychological problem, and we have now developed a definite point of view regarding this aspect.

The investigation of irradiation of the set which we mentioned above led to the obvious conclusion that irradiation of the set to a degree detectable by the method used in this case is not a universal phenomenon, but that, on the contrary, it is found only in certain cases, and it thus characterizes only the set of certain individuals. Moreover, when the state of irradiation has been determined in individual subjects, attention has been directed for a long time to its differential psychological nature. Unfortunately, however, we have not yet been able to examine it fully in special experimental investigations. Nevertheless, in the course of individual psychological investigation the aspects of irradiation of the set must not be ignored at the present time.

The same situation is found, of course, with the related problem of the generalization of the set. We found above that the aspect of generalization is a special aspect, with its own special objects and its own specific purpose, and it is of definite importance from the point of view of general theoretical psychological interests. At the same time, even with the small amount of material available today on this problem, its considerable differential psychological interest is clear enough. The problem of generalization of the set must therefore be specially investigated from the differential psychological point of view.

The evidence at present available on this problem shows that there is no shortage of interesting material for the study of the individual psychological features of different persons.

In Khachapuridze's book "Special Aspects of the Set in Children," cited above, we find evidence on the problem of the irradiation of the set in children. If we examine these facts from the differential psychological aspect, we find much of interest to the problem which we are now discussing. It must be remembered, however, that this investigation was completed at a time when the concept of generalization had not yet been developed, and it was then distantly associated with the concept of irradiation. For this reason, in the book just mentioned, we find no differential evidence on these two problems. Nevertheless, the results described in the book retain their importance even today.

These results may be summarized as follows:

A. Fixing experiments were carried out with preschool-age children in the haptic sphere (the ordinary wooden balls used in our experiments were presented as stimuli), while the critical experiments were performed in the optic sphere (two equal circles in a tachystoscope). The very first results which were obtained proved definitely that irradiation takes place. If measures were taken in the fixing experiments to fix the set "bigger on the right" haptically, in the critical experiments with the tachystoscope which followed immediately after the fixing experiments the circle on the right most frequently appeared bigger than the circle on the left; that is, assimilative illusions were found. However, this did not always happen in our experiments; in some cases, admittedly comparatively rarely, illusions of contrast occurred. On the basis of these experiments, repeatedly confirmed from different angles, the following results were obtained: assimilative illusions—42%, and contrast illusions—15%, that is, total number of cases of irradiation—57%. Hence we see that at preschool age the phenomenon of irradiation in the haptic and optic spheres is an undoubted fact.

B. With children of early school age the fixing exposures were given haptically as at preschool age. In the critical experiments, on the other hand, the subjects were shown a pair of equal circles on the screen, which were switched on for a moment and then switched off, so that the subject could see them clearly in order to compare them. What were the results of these experiments?

Of all the results available on this problem we shall choose those obtained with the largest number of subjects. Accordingly, we find that in this case there were 68% illusions of contrast and 21% assimilative illusions (the remaining 11% were correct responses; that is, equal critical objects were assessed correctly as equal). These figures show how quickly the number of illusions of contrast rises in school age. Admittedly, the number of assimilative perceptions in this case was not small (21%), but if we compare this figure with that observed at preschool age (42%) it is clear that the picture changes rapidly at this age, and this must undoubtedly be of great importance to the understanding of the course of development of the child's mind. This increase in the number of contrast illusions in the presence of irradiation points to changes taking place in the initial period of school life and indicates considerable development in the mind of the child, bringing it closer to the characteristics of adult mental life.

8. Constancy and Variability of the Fixed Set

We know that the process of extinction of the fixed set does not follow the same course in all cases and that because of this the set may be dynamic or static, plastic or coarse. However, our experimental investigations showed that people differ considerably from each other in that the type of extinction in some cases, depending on circumstances, changes frequently and does not remain constant, so that it is impossible to determine whether the particular individual, generally speaking, has a particular type of set. This conclusion naturally compels us to consider the general nature of the set: Is it something produced internally or is it entirely and exclusively determined by external conditions in which the particular subject has to live? This is a fundamental question, and its answer will largely explain the mechanisms of human behavior.

In order to answer this question we carried out experiments which were repeated after definite intervals of time (hours, days, weeks, months, and so on) without changing the experimental conditions at all. The results were meant to show whether the outcome of the experiments changed from one case to the other, and if so, in what conditions and to what degree.

The results showed that constancy of the set is not inevitable. There are some people in whom the set frequently changes, and there are others in whom the pattern of extinction of the fixed set always has the same series of stages.

We may conclude that constancy of the fixed set is not universal, but that some people exhibit types of variability of set.

Examination of these cases leads to a definite conclusion regarding the constancy of the set, namely, that the fixed set of a perfectly normal, healthy person remains constant in all cases. So far as the problem of variability is concerned, it may be concluded from a long series of observations that variability arises only in abnormal cases, which may be either temporary and transient or comparatively constant and stable. In the former we see rapid and superficial variations of the types of extinction of the set, while in the latter these variations are deeper and comparatively constant in character.

9. Stability and Lability of the Fixed Set

We mentioned above a new aspect of the fixed set which we described as its "stability." This is the ability of the set to remain capable of activity for a definite period of time.

In order to test this ability, we proceed as follows: As a result of a certain number of fixing experiments, we produce the corresponding fixed set. Then, after definite time intervals, the duration of which may be varied depending on the purpose of the experiment (hours, days, weeks), we carry out the critical experiments. In contrast to the experiments on constancy of the set, the fixing experiments are performed only at the beginning and are not thereafter repeated; only the critical experiments are repeated after the particular time intervals in which we are interested, and in each individual case they show what has happened to the fixed set—whether it has become extinguished or whether it still remains an active force.

We showed above that the fixed set, generally speaking, is stable. At the same time, however, we also pointed out that this property is of wide differential psychological significance. The set may be more or less stable or, on the other hand, it may be extremely labile. In this respect, people may differ considerably from each other, depending on various circumstances. The problem concerns the degree and the depth of stability. Hence, on the basis of experimental results, we may distinguish the following cases:

A. First, lability of the set is dependent on the time interval after which this set ceases to have any effect on the perception of critical objects. From this point of view, we must distinguish between fixed sets which lose their active force a few minutes or hours after their creation and those which lose it after days or weeks. Our experiments show that considerable differences are found between subjects, for whereas some are completely labile, completely unable to retain a fixed set even for a short time and to use it in case of need, others exhibit various degrees of stability. Some retain their set for weeks, others for months or even years. In brief, variability of subjects in this plane is of a high degree.

B. However, it is essential to examine the degree of constancy with which these persons retain this set. The results of our experiments show that this degree varies. Some people retain their set in the same form; the type of the fixed set does not change so long as it remains in force, and we see no signs of a gradual weakening of the strength of the fixed set—it remains invariably in the same form. In this case we could speak of the presence of a fixed set which could be defined as constant and stable. Finally, there are cases which are completely different—the set shows no constancy whatever. After certain time intervals, signs of variability appear; the set changes its type even while it remains in force. This may therefore be described as a variable–stable form of set, and several different degrees of this property may be found.

10. The Intermodal Nature of the Type of the Fixed Set

We have examined various aspects of the fixed set and we have found that each of them has its differential psychological application. We have not yet considered, however, a most important factor. We have as yet no direct evidence in support of the view that all these various aspects of the fixed set are essentially generalized properties, evidently extending to the organism as a whole, rather than specialized independent states of individual modalities. Otherwise, if the individual specific aspects of the set, such as its excitability, its dynamic or plastic nature, its constancy and stability, its irradiation and differentiation, were constant, invariable values regardless of the region in which they were found, we could then say that we were dealing with specific characteristics of the subject as a whole, and not those of his individual organs. Judging by what we already know about the set, we could solve this problem even without specially devised experiments. However, it seems desirable to turn to this question once again in order to obtain more precise material for our purpose.

And so, if we analyze the character of the fixed set in a subject from the point of view of every aspect known to us, in all the sensory fields which we possess, we may ask: What is the relationship between all these different aspects of manifestation of the set? If we investigate the special features of the set in a subject in the optic sphere, and then try to find out the state of the sets in the haptic and muscular spheres and what relationship they bear to each other, we shall obtain material suitable for providing the answer to our question.

We proceed as follows: It is advisable to carry out experiments with our subjects in three sensory modalities (in our case we usually select the optic, haptic, and motor fields), and in these fields we investigate the dynamicity, plasticity, constancy, stability, and excitability of the fixed set of each subject in order to find out the relationship between the results in each case—whether the individual modalities repeat each other or whether each is characterized by a set with its own individual features [4]. In brief, we must determine whether a particular type of fixed set is a constant feature of each particular subject or whether it may vary depending on the sensory modalities in which it arises.

In order to achieve this result, besides the usual measures we also used the following method: We extend the duration of the experiment by time intervals long enough to ensure that in each individual case the freedom of the results from the possible influence of irradiation may be guaranteed as far as possible. Typical results of these experiments are described below.

Of the 8 subjects whose results were specially studied at every stage of the experiment, 4 showed a definite pattern; their results were identical in all aspects of the set experimentally investigated. As an example, we cite Subject No. 1. He belonged to the group of inert-dynamic, weak, constant subjects, characterized by the lability and intermodally uniform excitability of the fixed set. This means that our subject exhibited the same type of extinction of the fixed set without change for 10 days. At first he gave a continuous series of illusions of contrast, and then, suddenly, without the usual intermediate forms, began to say that the objects shown to him were equal. He did this, however, not only in one particular field of perception, but in all three fields without exception. The fixed set of Subject No. 1 preserved its particular type of extinction in whatever sensory modality it developed.

The same picture was seen in relation to the remaining modification of the set; its excitability was the same in all directions. This was also true of its stability, despite the fact that when these subjects were investigated it was not possible to differentiate the stability of the set with respect to the degree of constancy.

The other 3 subjects showed the same picture of intermodal constancy of the fixed set, but they differed from Subject No. 1 in that he was of the type with a weak but coarse dynamic set, whereas the other 3, although likewise in the coarse, dynamic category, nevertheless showed definite stability of the set. The other subjects also had individual peculiarities which need not be discussed here. Admittedly, each of them gave his own particular pattern of fixed set, but they all resembled each other in that the fixed set invariably appeared in the same form in all the sensory modalities which we investigated.

The remaining group of subjects is of considerable interest. These were subjects who differed sharply from those we have just described in that the fixed set was variable, depending on which sensory modality was being investigated. Let us consider briefly what took place in these cases.

In contrast to the majority of subjects, 2 stood out particularly clearly, about whom it could be concluded that the pattern of extinction of the fixed set was unique. Each of them gave what seemed to be an original method of solving the problem—a method which differed radically from that used in previous cases. The characteristic feature of this method was the complete confusion of the picture and the vagueness of the main course of extinction of the set. Whereas in the preceding cases we invariably saw one definite method of extinction of the activity of the fixed set, in these subjects the pattern was abnormal and we saw the complete absence of any consistent order, of any more or less definite plan. The comparison of these two cases clearly illustrates this statement.

Subject No. 7 produced in the optic sphere a set characterized by its weak fixation, although it was inert and dynamic. In contrast, the picture was completely different in the haptic sphere and particularly in the muscular sphere. In the haptic sphere, our subject maintained the same picture of the fixed set as in the optic, but it was characterized by definite stability (the number of successive illusions of contrast here was not less than 13, whereas in the optic sphere it was not more than 5). A different state of affairs was found in the sphere of muscular sensation; here our subject was never able to free himself of a set once it had become fixed, however often the critical experiments were repeated. In this field, the set showed static fixation and could not be extinguished in conditions in which this usually occurs. The subject was unable to make the correct assessment of the equality of two weights, whereas the other subjects had no difficulty in doing so.

This same intermodal variability was also typical of the constancy of this subject's set. Whereas it was of the usual type in two sensory modalities—optic and muscular—it was completely different in the haptic sphere, where it was variable, appearing at the beginning as inert and static, but after about 2 days suddenly changing to a dynamic set. The lability of the set was also confused; although in the muscular field the subject always gave an illusion of contrast, that is, showed a stable–constant type of set, in the other modalities the opposite was seen. In the optic field, the set became extinguished after 2 days, and in the haptic sphere after only 1 day. Only the pattern of excitability (at least of its lower threshold) remained the same in all cases.

Hence, in general this subject revealed profound variability of the activity of the set depending on the sensory modalities through which it was produced. In short, in this case we have an intermodally variable fixed set.

The fixed set in Subject No. 8 was quite different and even more confused than the set in Subject No. 7. In the optic sphere, for example, this subject showed a plastic, but stable, form of set, but it remained fixed all the time and prevented all possibility of adequate perception. Consequently, although it was plastic, this did not prevent it from remaining a completely static fixed set.

The same picture was observed in the muscular sphere, with

the difference that the stable plastic set in this case was weak. However, the set was completely different in the haptic sphere, for although it remained plastic, the set in this sphere was dynamic. In this sensory sphere the subject freed himself comparatively easily from the influence of fixation and was able eventually to give a perfectly adequate assessment. Clearly, this form of set could hardly be described as constant, and indeed it changed its appearance continually, remaining comparatively constant only in the muscular sphere.

Finally, the stability of this set was variable: in the optic field it remained without visible change throughout the experiments, in the haptic field it was extinguished after the second day, and in the muscular field after the third day. Only from the point of view of excitability did the set in this subject remain approximately identical in all sensory modalities, and from the very beginning (after 3 to 5 exposures) it had the appearance of an intermodally inert, dynamic set.

Hence, it may be concluded that as a rule each normal subject has his own particular type of fixed set, which generally remains unchanged regardless of the sensory spheres involved in the process of its origin. It is found, however, that not all subjects belong to this principal, integral type, for there is a comparatively small number of persons who do not exhibit unity and conformity in the manifestations of their sets. In some spheres they present a completely different picture than in others. These are people with no inward singleness of purpose, people who are not rigidly set in a definite order, and frequently people characterized by internal conflict. At least we may say at this stage that, besides people with a normal makeup, others undoubtedly exist in whom the structure of the fixed set shows clear signs of abnormality

XIV. CONCLUSIONS

We have described the main facts in our possession concerning the problem of the set. What do they tell us?

The main conclusion is as follows: The development of conscious mental processes is preceded by a state which cannot in any degree be regarded as a nonmental, purely physiological state. We call this state "the set"—a state of preparedness for a definite activity, its onset depending on the presence of the following conditions: a need, actually felt by a particular organism, and an objective situation for the satisfaction of this need. These are the two essential and fully adequate conditions for the development of the set—without a need or an objective situation for its satisfaction, the set cannot be brought into activity, and in no case can some new and additional condition become necessary for the appearance of a set.

The set is a primary, integral, undifferentiated state. It is not a local process—rather it is a state characterized by irradiation and generalization. Despite this fact, on the basis of the results of experimental investigation of the set we may define it from different points of view.

First, it has been found that the set in its initial phase usually appears as a diffuse, undifferentiated state, and before it can obtain a more definite and differentiated form, the influence of the repeated action of a situation is necessary. At some stage of the action of this repeated stimulus, the set becomes fixed, and from then on we have a definite form of fixed set.

The set is produced in response to the action of situations, which may be differentiated into quantitative or qualitative relationships, on a subject. No significant difference is found between these two cases, and the principles governing the activity of the set in both cases remain the same in their essential features.

These principles are manifested in different directions, and they characterize different aspects of the state of the set in a subject. We have seen that fixation of the set, like its differentiation, does not take place uniformly quickly (degree of excitability of the set). We have also seen that extinction of the set takes place in accordance with a definite rule: It passes through a series of stages, and only after this does it reach a stage of extinction. In this case, however, outward signs of individual variation appear; with regard to completeness of extinction we may distinguish static and dynamic sets, and from the point of view of the stages of extinction, plastic and coarse sets. It should be noted that the constancy of a fixed set is not always the same; it may be primarily labile or primarily stable. The same may be said regarding its typological constancy. From this point of view, we may distinguish constant and variable sets.

Hence, it is clear that the set may be defined from different points of view, and its distinctive properties must be qualified from different aspects. We have seen that in man a whole sphere of activity exists which precedes his ordinary conscious mental activity, and the study of this sphere is undoubtedly of great scientific interest, for without a special analysis of it there can be no hope of obtaining an adequate understanding of human psychology.

Our next task is to study the problem of the set in animals, and if we find that the set exists in some form or other in animals this will present us with both the opportunity and necessity of seeking specific forms of activity of the set in man.

Set in Animals

1. Enunciation of the Problem

We have seen that the main conditions for the appearance of a set in man are the presence of a need and the presence of a situation for its satisfaction. Since there is nothing specific and exclusively human about these conditions, we may naturally ask whether a set may be created in animals. We have no reason to assume that a set toward corresponding activity may arise on the basis of need and situation only in man. On the contrary, since in man consciousness plays a pre-eminent role, and since in animals it is not evident, we may suppose that the set in animals would be particularly important.

In order to demonstrate conclusively that sets exist in animals, the solution to the problem should first be sought experimentally. We now have considerable experience with the experimental study of human sets. We shall, of course, make use of this fact and try to devise a method of studying animals which resembles as closely as possible our ordinary and well-tried method of investigation of the set in man. Admittedly, in these experiments we make use of the fact that the subject can speak, but the participation of language in this case is not of fundamental importance, and it can easily be replaced without adverse effect on the results of the experiment. We can use the results of these experiments to solve conclusively the problem of the presence of sets in animals as well as to determine their relationship to our findings in man.

We have now investigated the problem of sets in birds (especially in the domestic hen), in albino rats and, finally, in monkeys. Although the method is basically the same in all cases, it must of necessity vary depending on the purpose and conditions of the experiment; therefore, besides describing the results of the experiment, in each case we shall also describe the method in detail.

Experiments by the method of the fixed set were first carried out on lower monkeys by N. Yu. Voitonis.* These experiments gave positive results. However, we shall not dwell on them here, since they were not performed in our laboratory and their results were used by Voitonis in connection with a wider examination of the problem.

I shall consider in greater detail investigations carried out in my own Institute under my own observation and direction.

2. Experiments with Hens [114]

The problem was first studied in the domestic hen: Can we speak of a set in hens, and if so, can it be fixed and what is its course?

In order to answer these questions, we gave a hen food consisting of wheat grains scattered over the surface of a board divided into two halves — one half dark and the other half light. The grains on the light half were firmly glued to the surface and could not be pecked off; nothing interfered with their removal from the darker half. The board was given to the hen so that it could peck two or three times, and then it was removed so that the food could no longer be seen. This was repeated several times (that is, as a fixing experiment). Next we proceeded to the critical experiments: The hen was given the same board, but this time both halves were the same color and the food was scattered freely over its surface. Depending on the set fixed in the preliminary experiments, the hen pecked either on the right half or on the left.

3. The Set in Hens

The results of these experiments showed conclusively that sets may exist in hens, and that as a result of repeated fixing experiments, these sets can be fixed to a greater or lesser degree. It should be noted, however, that in this case the fixation of the set is marked by certain distinctive features, determined by our experimental conditions. In experiments with human subjects we know that fixation of the set is easily accomplished; two or three exposures as a rule are sufficient to exceed the lower threshold of fixation. With hens, however, the minimal number of fixing exposures may be as many as 20.

In hens, of course, we have a phenomenon of a distinctive type. It is possible that the difficulty of fixation of the set in this case is primarily dependent on difficulty of differentiation. When

*N. Yu. Voitonis, "Forms of Manifestation of Sets in Animals and Especially in Monkeys," Psikhologiya 3 (1944).

receiving the fixing exposures, the hen must differentiate the developing set so that ultimately it can fix it. Hence, it can be concluded that although sets undoubtedly exist in hens, fixation of these sets takes much longer than in man. The reason for this may be that the set in birds is relatively undifferentiated, and that a large number of exposures is required to ensure final and complete differentiation.

A further scrutiny of these experiments reveals yet another special feature of the set. We know that in quantitative experiments with human subjects the illusions are predominantly those of contrast, and assimilative illusions are comparatively rare. In experiments with hens, however, this is not so. The number of assimilative illusions is large, and the conditions of their appearance are seen much more clearly than in experiments with man. In the experiments with hen No. 1, for example, these illusions accounted for 85% of the total number — a much higher figure than for the same experiments with human subjects. In man, however, we saw clearly that illusions develop only in certain cases, namely, when the fixing experiments do not differ greatly from each other, or, at least, before the set has become adequately fixed. This conclusion, which I first discovered as the result of observations on the activity of the fixed set in man, is seen much more frequently in experiments with hens than in in experiments with human subjects.

So far as illusions of contrast are concerned, as a rule the more firmly fixed the set, the more frequently these appear in hens. This confirms once again that in these experiments we were actually dealing with a set, that is, the phenomenon which we first encountered in man.

Hence, it is clear that if suitable conditions are present, sets may develop in hens and they may become fixed. Naturally this possibility is limited, and sets develop much more slowly than in man, but it must be assumed that these characteristics will produce specific conditions for the manifestation of assimilative illusions, the number of which in these experiments far exceeded those found in experiments with human subjects.

However, the same circumstances lead subsequently to the more frequent appearance of illusions of contrast. After the stage of assimilation, they gradually become more stable and eventually they completely supplant the stage of assimilation.

One further feature of the process of fixation of the set stands out much more clearly in these experiments than in experiments with human subjects. In the course of the experiments, hen No. 3

began to show one characteristic feature — after 10 days of daily experiments, this bird's behavior changed sharply and it ceased altogether to react to the experimental conditions. As soon as the experimental board with the food was presented, the hen turned away from it and continued to stand motionless until the experimenter went away. In this way the hen refused to eat for $2\frac{1}{2}$ days; nothing whatever was given to the hen to eat outside the experiment. Nevertheless, the bird continued to behave in this way, absolutely refusing to eat in experimental conditions. On the third day, during the fixing exposure, the bird hesitantly began to approach the experimental board and to peck at the positive half (that is, the half from which the grain could be pecked), but when, after 29 fixing exposures, the hen was shown the "critical" board, it stood as if petrified, holding its head up high and standing motionless for several seconds. . .it then turned away and moved off clucking.

Obviously, the number of exposures in the experiment with this hen was limited. On the other hand, when this number grew too large, something unexpected happened: The hen became unable to react or, more accurately, refused completely to react, and even after starving for 3 days it could not overcome this state of inactivity. In this case, we were undoubtedly dealing with a specific state, out of which arose a phenomenon similar to the "satiety" which was examined in such detail by Kurt Lewin [2].

This example shows the existence of a normal level, which, if exceeded, leads to the total collapse of the animal's activity. This normal level may perhaps coincide with the optimal number of presentations for the particular animal. The question of the optimum in this case is reflected by the sharply defined forms not usually found at the higher levels of development. This does not mean, however, that they can be ignored here.

In these experiments we obtain material relevant to the solution of the problem of the fixability and stability of the fixed set in hens. So far as the first of these is concerned, it was found that a fixed set in a hen remains in force only for 2 or 3 critical exposures. So far as the stability of this set is concerned, it was found to remain constant for only 24 hours. This does not mean, however, that it cannot last longer than this. In fact, it lasted about 3 days, but in a variable form; that is, it remained in force but became labile in its manifestations. This process of its regressive development was not complete until after 3 days.

Hence, it is clear that in hens, sets become active, differentiated, and fixed. However, it is equally clear that these processes are much more primitive than in man; sets in hens are evidently relatively undifferentiated from the very beginning, and before some degree of differentiation can be achieved, followed by fixation in this form, a comparatively large number of fixing exposures is required. Nevertheless, this fixation is unstable and quickly disappears after 2 to 3 critical experiments. If it is not constantly maintained, it remains in its unchanged form for only 24 hours, and for 2 to 3 days in a variable form.

I. SET IN ALBINO RATS

1. Experimental Method

A small cage with an entrance on one side and two exits on the opposite side, one covered with light gray cardboard and the other with much darker cardboard, was used. The rat was placed in the cage, and when it came out through the darker exit it received food. If it came out through the lighter exit it received nothing. After a certain number of experiments, both exits were covered with cardboard of the same shade. We know that after a certain number of fixing exposures, the two shades of cardboard begin to appear different to the animals; one appears lighter and the other darker. Assuming that the rat develops a set toward passing through the dark exit, in the critical experiment it will try to pass through the exit which appears darker.

In a second series of experiments, the pieces of gray cardboard were replaced by pieces on which were drawn circles differing considerably in size. In the first series of fixing experiments, the rat became accustomed to pass through the exit with the larger circle; as soon as it entered the cage it ran out through this exit and received food. In the critical experiment it was able to run from the cage by both exits.

2. Experimental Results

We will now discuss some of the results of these experiments. The first question which we must answer is: Does a set become fixed in the albino rat or not? In experiments carried out by our collaborator N. Chrelashvili, who was the first to study these problems, it was found that, as in the experiments with the hens,

TABLE XIII

Fixing experiments	Number of critical experiments	Illusions of contrast		Assimilative illusions	
		Absolute number	%	Absolute number	%
1 – 137	39	6	15	25	64
137 – 190	38	34	89	4	10

the set became fixed only comparatively late, and not until the 35th, 50th, or 65th exposures did isolated illusions begin to appear.

Later, as is clear from Table XIII, until the 137th fixing experiment assimilative illusions were predominant. This means that assimilation takes place here predominantly in the initial period of the experiment, before the set has had the opportunity to become finally fixed. Naturally, therefore, after a large number of exposures of the fixing object (137 to 190), illusions of contrast began to appear (89%). Admittedly, assimilation still continued to appear, but only very rarely and exceptionally (10%).

The same phenomenon was observed in these experiments as in those with the hens; namely, when the number of exposures increased appreciably, for example, after 6 to 9 critical exposures, the rate at which the rats worked became slower, they began to hesitate before choosing, they reacted much more slowly, and finally, their reactions lost all purposiveness. In the hens, in similar conditions, complete refusal to take part in the experiments was sometimes observed. Admittedly, this did not happen with the rats; nevertheless, it is clear that a phenomenon of the same category as with the hens also took place. The fact that "satiety" was really concerned here was proved by the results of slightly modified fixing experiments. When the rat received constantly changing stimuli rather than always the same, and the relationship between the fixing objects did not remain constant, it was found that the rat continued to react stably and for a long period; illusions of contrast remained in force during 20 to 25 critical exposures, and the pattern of rapid and decisive reactions was maintained throughout.

It is interesting that here, in experiments with constant and changing fixing exposures, the results obtained were not absolutely identical. When the rat was exposed to the action of always the same fixing exposures, the set thus produced was not particularly stable and remained in force only for 6 to 9 critical experiments, after which, clear signs of hesitation and slowing of the tempo of reactions, as well as a decrease in the purposiveness of the activity of the rat, were observed.

A different picture was seen when varying fixing exposures were used. For example, when the fixing objects were varied, the illusion developing in these conditions persisted throughout a long series of exposures. An illusion of contrast still appeared even after 20 to 25 critical exposures.

Attention must be drawn to another distinctive feature of a set arising during the action of varying fixing exposures; it could be transposed into a series of analogous relationships. What is meant is as follows: If a fixed set is produced to a series of relationships between degrees of illumination, the set can be transposed to another series of relationships not found in the fixing experiments. However, these relationships must not differ very considerably from those of the fixing experiments, for in cases in which the fixing exposures remained unchanged, that is, when the set was fixed by the repeated action of the same fixing stimulus, transposition hardly ever took place.

Interesting results were observed after application of series of varying fixing exposures. When a series of 10 exposures was applied, an illusion of contrast developed which remained unchanged to the end (a coarse static set). When, on the other hand, the number of exposures was reduced to 4 or 5, a different picture was obtained, and besides illusions of contrast, assimilative illusions were evoked, and they were more numerous than the former.

As far as experiments to study the stability of the set are concerned, they gave the following results. If a rat in which a corresponding fixed set had previously been evoked received a series of critical objects on the day after the fixing experiments, it was found that the fixed set continued to operate, lasting, as a rule, for another 24 to 48 hours. Consequently, the fixed set in albino rats is stable for 2 to 3 days.

II. SET IN MONKEYS

1. Experimental Method

Since no anthropoids are kept at present in the Tbilisi Zoological Gardens, our experiments on set had to be restricted to lower monkeys. Our colleague N. G. Adamashvili carried out these experiments on two capuchin monkeys (Vova, aged 8 years, and Vivi, aged 2.5 years). The method was the same in principle as the ordinary experiments on fixed sets. In one series of experiments, carried out only with Vova, the monkey received repeated fixing exposures consisting of pairs of meals, one small and the other large. After a series of such exposures, the monkey was then given two meals of equal size in the critical experiments.

Besides these, a second series of experiments was carried out – initially with Vova, and then with Vivi, who had not taken part in the experiments of the first series.

For the first $1^1/_2$ months, training experiments were carried out on the monkey to accustom it to react differentially to baits of the same and different sizes. When the monkey received baits of different sizes it took the larger one, and the smaller one was then immediately removed, whereas if identical baits were presented the monkey chose one after the other. As a result of these training experiments, the monkey chose only the larger of two unequal baits and left the smaller one untouched. So far as equal baits are concerned, the monkey took them one after the other and ate them.

After the training experiments, the fixing experiments began. The exposures continued long enough for the monkey to be able to take both baits if presented with baits of equal sizes.

2. The Presence of a Fixed Set in Monkeys

Although the preceding experiments clearly showed that sets undoubtedly occur in monkeys, and are equally accessible to experimental investigation as in man, nevertheless the question arises whether in the experiments with monkeys we were in fact dealing with sets or whether, on the other hand, the phenomena observed had nothing in common with sets in man.

Let us first consider what took place in these experiments. When the monkey received two bowls of food (in our fixing experiments) it was accustomed to choosing the larger bait. In the critical experiments in which two bowls containing the same amount of food were presented, in most cases the monkey chose the bowl on the side on which in the fixing experiments the smaller bowl had been placed. From all signs, this was a case of an illusion of volume, which evidently determined the monkey's behavior. We know that this illusion is based on the set fixed in the preceding experiments. Consequently, it may be assumed that in this case we were dealing with our usual illusion of the fixed set.

The correctness of this conclusion will be obvious if it is remembered that as a rule, similar phenomena also occurred in experiments with human subjects during the investigation of their fixed sets. Further confirmation is afforded by the fact that the same phenomenon also takes place in other animals (in hens and rats). Nevertheless, it would not be superfluous to examine all the most probable alternative solutions of the problem facing the monkey.

In the first place we must ask ourselves whether the reactions of the animal in the critical experiments were the result of the reinforcement, fixation, and mechanization of the behavioral acts of the animal during the fixing experiments. This hypothesis, of course, can apply only to the assimilative illusions developing in the monkeys in these experimental conditions. So far as illusions of contrast are concerned, since they are opposite in direction to the fixing reactions of the animal, this hypothesis cannot of course concern them. In this case, illusions opposite to those which have been reinforced, fixed, and mechanized could hardly take place.

However, if this is impossible in relation to illusions of contrast, it must undoubtedly be accepted in relation to assimilative illusions; we know that both these illusions are essentially phenomena of the same category. Nevertheless, let us try to assume that assimilative illusions are independent phenomena, having nothing in common in this case with illusions of contrast. Can we not suppose that in this case they must be interpreted as the result of the fixation and mechanization of the fixing exposures? Such an interpretation of these reactions would be quite natural, and would be entirely justified if, in the case of assimilative illusions, there were no doubt whatever that we were dealing with the repetition of exactly the same reactions as in the fixing experiments.

But is this so? Analysis of the assimilative reactions arising in these cases shows that they were of a third type. Firstly, in this case the assimilative reactions arose without any hesitation, immediately after the critical exposures. We have no direct grounds for asserting that they are the result of the fixing exposures and not of the simple fixation and mechanization of these reactions. Accordingly, all these cases may be ignored. On the other hand, we had two other cases in which we undoubtedly were dealing with a new, adequate, but not mechanized reaction, repeated only because it was fixed. These reactions were characterized by the fact that in one instance, reaction was preceded by an obvious period of hesitation, while in the other a similar period of hesitation was observed immediately after completion of the reaction. A mere glance at the structure of these reactions is enough to show that they were not random but that, on the contrary, in both instances they were selective reactions. It would be completely impossible to find another explanation of the fact that hesitation was present before and after the reaction.

Hence, we see that the hypothesis that the reactions of the animal could be attributed to fixation of mechanized behavior does not rest on a firm enough basis.

There is another possible explanation: The monkey's behavior is determined by the fact that in the fixing experiments it was accustomed to react to stimulation "from the left." Its reactions were therefore simply reactions of habituation to a definite orientation in space. However, we have only to remember the distinctive structure of the reactions of the animal to be convinced that this hypothesis is invalid. The observations showed that the animal's reactions were accompanied by periods of hesitation. If these reactions had been simply a series of successive habitual movements, no hesitation would have taken place. This conclusion must be regarded as proved if it is remembered that in these experiments we observed not only assimilative illusions, but also, and more frequently, illusions of contrast, which were always opposite to the habitual direction.

It might be thought that the direction of the monkey's actions was always determined by the limb which happened to be active at the particular moment: If it was the right limb, it would be directed toward the food on the right; if the left, the monkey would try to grasp the food on the left side. This suggestion was justified in several cases, and in nearly all the initial stages of the experiments. However, when a short time had elapsed and the set had become sufficiently fixed, no trace of this remained: The monkey in these cases as a rule gave reactions corresponding perfectly to the meaning of the fixed set.

Finally, as Adamashvili points out, in some cases a definite rhythm of behavior was produced in the animal under the influence of exercise, and it followed this rhythm. It might be supposed that some rhythm of this type was present in our experiments. However, the mere enunciation of this question is sufficient to reject it categorically. There is no doubt that in our experiments there were no conditions for the development of any particular rhythm of action on the part of the monkey; our critical experiments had nothing which could justify the assumption of a rhythmic sequence of these experiments.

To sum up, we have no grounds for suggesting that the animal's reactions — whether of contrast or assimilation — were acts of an accidental character, unrelated to the preceding fixing exposures. We must conclude that the acts of the monkey were nothing more than the result of our usual fixing illusions, arising in this case just in the same way as in our other experimental animals. In this case, also, we may speak of illusions of the set.

When the monkey received food, let us say on the right side, in a series of fixing experiments, while in the critical experiments, in which two equal baits were offered, it took the bait on the left side, this means that the bait on the left appeared bigger than the one on the right (illusion of contrast), so that the animal hastened to take it. In other experiments, in certain conditions, the bait on the left side may appear more attractive (bigger in size), and this may lie at the basis of the converse phenomenon — the assimilative illusion.

This observation shows conclusively that in certain conditions the same illusions of sets arise in monkeys as in the other animals we have investigated and also in man.

3. Fixed Sets in Monkeys

We must now take a closer look at these reactions of the monkey.

In the first place it must be stressed that in monkeys, just as in man or other animals, we found both types of reactions based on sets — assimilative and contrast. Moreover, the principles governing the appearance of these illusions in this case were the same as in the other cases; namely, assimilative illusions develop more frequently when the difference between the fixing stimuli is slight, and also when the fixing experiments are few in number. This principle, familiar to us from experiments with human subjects, is confirmed sufficiently clearly in animals and, in particular, in monkeys.

It is clear from Table XIV that when distinguishing between baits differing in size by amounts varying from 0.5 to 1.00 mm, assimilative illusions appeared almost exclusively (from 75% to 90.3%) in the monkeys. However, when the difference was increased beyond this limit, the situation changed and the number of contrast illusions

TABLE XIV

Difference in size	Assimilative illusions	Illusions of contrast	Equality
0. 5 mm	75.0	8.3	16.6
1. 0 "	90.3	6.5	3.2
1. 5 "	61.7	28.5	9.4
3. 0–6. 0	47.0	45.0	8.0

increased. When the difference between the fixing stimuli reached 3 to 6 mm, the number of contrast illusions became equal to the number of assimilative illusions. Later, as we know from other findings, the contrast illusions began to predominate clearly over the number of assimilative illusions, and finally, the latter ceased to appear entirely.

The same picture was seen when the number of fixing exposures was varied. In this case (Table XV) the maximal number of assimilative illusions fell after 1 to 3 fixing exposures, while if this number was increased, the number of contrast illusions rose considerably, while the assimilative illusions became less frequent.

We thus find that the principles governing the development of assimilative and contrast illusions in the monkey are basically the same as those in man. We find that with a very slight increase in the number of fixing exposures (the optimal number must evidently be considered to be 2), and also when the difference between the fixing objects is very slight, monkeys develop an assimilative illusion, whereas with an increase in the number of fixing exposures and also in the quantitative difference between them, illusions of contrast begin to develop, and the further this process is taken, the greater the predominance of illusions of contrast over assimilation.

If we now turn to other aspects of the fixed sets of monkeys, the first question to consider is the degree of their excitability. A

TABLE 15

Number of fixing exposures	Assimilative illusions	Illusions of contrast	Equality
1	9.4	6.2	84.4
2.3	16.1	25.9	58.1
5	10.0	40.0	50.0
10.5	15.0	45.0	40.0

series of experiments with two monkeys yielded results from which the excitability of their fixed sets could be determined. It was found that in some cases, a set was fixed in a monkey after a series of exposures, but that in other cases, despite the fact that the number of fixing exposures was the same or even higher than before, no fixation of the set whatever took place. This strange instability of the excitability of the set in monkeys was also reflected by the fact that sometimes the set showed no signs of fixation, even after the number of fixing exposures ordinarily just sufficient to produce fixation.

This variability of the excitability of the fixed set is a very characteristic feature of the monkeys which we tested, and possibly it is not peculiar to them alone. However, where excitability is an obvious fact, it seems to be an index of high sensitivity. In experiments with monkeys we found that one or two exposures were often enough to produce adequate fixation of the set.

Hence, we may conclude that the coefficient of excitability of the set in monkeys may admittedly be very low (1 or 2 exposures), but in general it is an exceedingly variable figure, varying from case to case within very wide limits, extending down to zero.

This fact makes us dubious of the possibility of a high degree of stability of the fixed set in our monkeys. This property is measured, as we know, by the data of a continuous sequence of contrast illusions. We found that in the monkey Vova, twice there was a series of six illusions and twice a series of nine illusions of contrast appeared, whereas in the remaining four instances we found only isolated illusions. Approximately the same results were observed with the other monkey (Vivi). This suggests that generally speaking we could not assume the presence of a firmly fixed set in these monkeys. Like its excitability, its stability is not a constant value in the monkey — it changes from case to case, and the true basis of these changes is certainly of sufficient importance to warrant special investigation.

We must now examine the process of extinction of the fixed set in monkeys. For this purpose we made use of the usual method of repeated application of critical stimuli until the fixed set was extinguished and replaced by a new set more adequate to the fresh conditions. The results of these experiments are described below.

Without going into detail in describing these results, it may be said that our monkeys, in our experimental conditions, very rarely reached the stage of complete extinction of the fixed set. It was clear everywhere that the sign of variability, which was demonstrated in these animals in other cases also (for example, during the investigation of excitability), is a very distinctive and characteristic feature. It is clear from the results obtained, that whereas at a particular moment 2 or 3 critical exposures were sufficient to produce extinction of the corresponding fixed set, at another time this would not be sufficient for this purpose, and a much larger number of exposures was needed; otherwise the same fixed set would not be suppressed.

Hence, we may conclude that in our monkeys the sign of the dynamic character of the fixed set showed a high degree of variability.

So far as the plasticity of the set in these monkeys is concerned, this is a highly problematical value. In one monkey extinction of the fixed set was never seen; the animal never once reacted to the critical stimuli as equal. If we could guarantee that the conditions were corresponding, and the monkey proceeded to this last phase of the experiments, we would then obtain an approximately identical picture in both monkeys, and we would then say that the fixed set in these animals was not so lacking in plasticity as might appear at first glance. Nevertheless, even in these conditions it could not be said that we were in fact dealing with a plastic, fixed set, because in that case we would observe the successive unfolding of all the stages or phases of the process of extinction of the fixed set.

In brief, we find that the fixed set in monkeys is distinguished by low plasticity, variability, and dynamicity.

Finally, the results of special experiments undertaken to study the stability of the fixed set in monkeys were as follows: If a set was fixed in monkeys, it remained active for a fairly long time. In some cases it still remained fully active one week after the day of fixation. It was found, however, that the sign of variability, characteristic of the set in monkeys in other cases, was also characteristic here. It was frequently found that the monkey became unable to act in the direction evidently firmly fixed by the set, whereas another time, on the contrary, we were struck by the activity displayed in this direction.

III. GENERAL CHARACTERISTICS OF THE SET IN ANIMALS

The following general conclusions may be drawn from the results of investigations of sets in animals:

1. The set is not a specifically human characteristic. Experiments have shown that it is a characteristic property of all the animals which we have investigated. Moreover, the ability to react to the environment in the form of a particular set is the most characteristic property of any living organism, whatever its stage of development. It is the most primitive, yet at the same time the most fundamental, form of reaction of the living organism to external environmental conditions.

2. Analysis of the set in the animals which we investigated shows clearly that at the early stages of its development the set is more or less diffuse in character, and before becoming fixed it must pass through several phases of differentiation. In particular, in the animals which we investigated – in hens, rats, and monkeys – it appeared more frequently in this undifferentiated form than it did in man.

This comparatively low degree of differentiation of the set is reflected in the fact that in the animals which we investigated, the set was inconstant in the forms of its manifestation. Whereas, for example, at one moment it appeared as a definite type of activity, at another moment it could appear in a completely different form – it could disappear completely, or it could be highly active.

Set In Man

I. THE PROBLEM OF OBJECTIVIZATION

1. Two Spheres of Action on Man

If we ask ourselves what is the specific chracteristic of man distinguishing him from other living creatures, our first thought will probably be that it is speech, and we shall say that man is blessed with the power of speech whereas other living creatures are completely without it. Another question which we may ask is: Is this faculty a secondary phenomenon, based on some other phenomenon of more fundamental importance than speech itself? Without going into this question in detail, we can state that there is nothing, with the exception of the world around us, which can influence and determine our behavior so much as speech.

We could express the same idea differently; we could state that there is nothing more characteristic of man than the fact that his external environment influences him in two ways — directly, by sending him a series of stimuli directly acting upon him, and indirectly, through verbal symbols which, while possessing no true meaning of their own, represent to us certain forms of stimulation. Man perceives either the direct influence of the processes going on around him or the influence of verbal symbols representing these processes in a specific form. Whereas an animal's behavior is determined entirely by the influence of the surrounding world, man is not always directly under the control of this external reality; more often, he reacts to its phenomena only after he has assimilated them into consciousness, only after he has grasped their meaning. It is obvious that this is a very essential characteristic of man, which may be responsible for his ascendancy over other living creatures.

What is this faculty upon which this human characteristic is based? From what we already know of man, we naturally form some idea of the role which this set may play in this case. Therefore, our purpose must now be to determine the role and the place of this concept in human life.

If it is true that our behavior, which has developed as a result of the direct influence of the external environment on us, is based on sets, then what happens in a different plane — the plane of verbal reality, represented in words? Do our sets play some part here, or is this sphere of our activity constructed on completely different foundations?

2. The Problem of Attention

Before solving this problem, we must use as our starting point the problem of attention or, more precisely, the possibility of the act of attention, especially the problem of the comprehension of this act. It is usually considered that attention is essentially selective in character, that it enables us to select from a series of impressions acting upon us a particular one and to concentrate on it so that it can be presented with maximal clarity and precision.

However, a superficial glance at this definition is sufficient to demonstrate that it is essentially much too vague. Moreover, the definition itself invites a series of questions, without the preliminary solution of which it is impossible to select any one of the possible definitions of attention.

First, is it necessary for us to direct attention toward something before it can become an object of our consciousness? Before we can direct attention to something, must it have been given to us already to some degree? But for this to be possible, that is, for it to have been given to us, must we not previously have turned our attention to it In principle, of course, the question of the degree of concentration of attention is unimportant, and the problem which concerns us is the possibility of the primary concentration of attention, irrespective of the degree to which it may take place.

It thus becomes clear that the usual definition of attention does not give us a clear idea of, nor help us in any way to understand, what it is that we mean by attention. These remarks, of course, apply to the most widely used definition of this concept. But other definitions exist. Can the same be said about them?

I consider that the basic idea which concerns us here is common to all the known attempts to define attention. In all definitions the main function of attention is considered to be the same, namely, to increase the degree of lucidity and clarity of the developing idea, and if these definitions differ from each other in some respect, in any case it is not in this. Accordingly, so far as the basic idea of the existing definitions of our concept is concerned, we can be content with the foregoing.

If we accept this definition, the thought may arise that it is not concerned with any single process. Rather it may be supposed that we are concerned with the dual presentation of the same phenomenon. Impressions acting upon us are perceived in two ways: on the one hand, as phenomena not accompanied by acts of our attention, and on the other, as the same phenomena, but this time mediated by these acts. Consequently, we may perceive a series of phenomena, but without imagining them clearly and lucidly; if our attention is active, we experience them clearly and lucidly. This does not mean, of course, that the activity of our attention is weak in the first case and strong in the second. In the first case no activity of our attention whatever is present.

Consequently, in some cases our thought works and, in particular, perceives a series of phenomena, but without any participation of our attention; that is, it perceives phenomena which are vague and imprecise. In the ordinary definition of attention it is suggested that this may take place, that phenomena completely devoid of clarity and lucidity may occur in consciousness. But it is hardly logical to accept the presence in man of such phenomena which gain nothing from the fact that they have become mental experiences, that they remain the same as before for the subject, that is, something foreign, unknown, and nonexistent.

We must evidently accept that if such mental experiences exist, they are always accompanied by a certain degree of "consciousness," regardless of whether in these cases we can speak of the participation of attention or not. Otherwise, there will be no reason to consider that we are in fact dealing with mental experiences.

The suggestion may be made that the traditional understanding of attention may be based on the unrecognized thought that the working of the human mind can be dissociated into two different planes, one of which does not require the participation of attention, while the other does. In both cases, moreover, there is no doubt about the presence of lucidity and clarity. Our object now is to demonstrate that these planes of the working of consciousness in fact exist and that this must be taken into consideration before mental life can be understood at the various stages of its development.

3. Two Planes of Working of the Human Mind

What are these planes of working of our minds about which we are speaking?

Until now it must be admitted that the need to use these two planes of working of the human mind has not been considered in psychology as clearly as it should have been. However, with the scientific recognition of many of the phenomena of mental life has come the need to make assumptions which, although essentially incorrect, have nevertheless given clues to a number of factors, the study of which could in the future reveal the true nature of these phenomena.

So that a clear idea could be obtained of these planes of working of consciousness, we tried to analyze one of the most usual cases of human behavior. Let us assume that a man wakes up and turns to his usual act of behavior; he begins to dress, puts on his shoe, and begins to tie it, when he suddenly finds that he is not making progress and that something is obstructing him. In this case, a dual relationship to this phenomenon can be contemplated: Either the subject does not pay attention to this comparatively unimportant phenomenon but continues to dress all the same, or at this moment he ceases the act of putting on his shoe, pauses for some time, and begins to fix his attention on the shoe to find out the reason for this unexpected interference. He must do this before he can remove this cause and finish his essential behavioral act.

This elementary example is one of the most usual cases, such as may be described at any step in our life, and it may be assumed that the whole of human life is largely constructed of series of such processes. We must examine it more closely so we can see that in this case we are dealing with an undoubtedly important phenomenon, shedding light on the true nature of human mental life.

In this comparatively elementary and usual act of our behavior, we may discern the presence of two separate planes of activity of the mind — the plane of "impulsive" activity, and the plane of "objectivated" activity. We must now devote our attention to the analysis of these two planes in order to obtain a clear idea of what we are discussing.

A. The Plane of Impulsive Behavior

Turning to the first of these, that is, the plane of "impulsive" behavior, we find that its specific psychological feature is the direct inclusion of the subject and of his acts in the continuous process of behavior. In order to obtain a clearer picture of the specific features of this impulsive behavior, the instinctive activity of an animal, or habitual, mechanised human activity, may serve as an example.

In these cases there is an act of reflection on the appropriate elements of the outside world, which the subject reflects upon not as an integral whole, not in all its details, but only with respect to that particular part of it directly related to the purposes of the behavior. They are reflected upon clearly enough to become operative factors in the subject's behavior. The hen, for example, must notice the presence of the grains in order to start pecking. For this act of behavior to be stimulated, there is no need to make a detailed examination of these grains; provided the hen notices them, it can start pecking. This is quite sufficient to keep the hen alive.

If, on the other hand, we turn to our example of getting up in the morning, a man must be able to choose his clothes or shoes from the surrounding objects and to perceive them clearly enough to be able to dress himself. This is absolutely essential for him, and it is quite adequate in the ordinary conditions of his daily life. Any goal-directed activity must include the selection of influences acting on the subject, the concentration of appropriate mental energy on them, and their sufficiently clear reflection in his mind. Otherwise, activity arising in these conditions would be nothing more than a chaotic series of individual acts bearing no relation either to the subject's goal or to the nature of the external situation in which they took place.

Despite the fact that in this case we are also dealing with the choice of influences acting on a subject and with the concentration of mental energy on these agents, and also with their clear reflection in the mind, there are still no true grounds for assuming the participation of attention in these acts. Besides images of perception and individual forms of activity included in the process of impulsive behavior, the phenomena of consciousness are also characterized by a special feature which excludes any idea that acts of attention may be responsible for them: They arise and operate only to be replaced quickly and without any delay by subsequent acts which they themselves stimulate, and these in turn continue the same process. They play the role of separate links in the whole chain of behavior — the role of signals stimulating the next steps in the process of behavior. They have no independent value; they do not exist alone outside this role, or separately from the process of behavior in which they are continuously included. Impulsive behavior is completely dependent on impulses arising from a combination of internal and external environmental conditions — completely and utterly dependent on the actual situation surrounding the subject at the particular moment. In his acts of impulsive behavior, the subject is the slave of the environmental conditions acting upon him at the time.

The question arises: What is it in this case, if it is not the specific faculty customarily called attention, which determines these processes of selection of those influences which are related to the purposes of our behavior, the concentration of "mental energy" on them, and, as a result, their clear-enough perception in consciousness? This problem is completely insoluble in ordinary psychology, which indiscriminately disregards those processes taking place in us which are still unknown to the old, traditional science. In the light of our theory of set, this problem is not particularly difficult to solve. We know that, according to this theory, whenever a certain need arises, the living organism or, more accurately, the subject strives to establish a certain relationship to the external environment — to the situation for satisfaction of this need — so that the need which has arisen may in fact be satisfied. For its part, as the situation for the satisfaction of the present need, the environment acts directly, not on individual mental or physiological processes taking place in the organism feeling this need, but on the living organism as a whole, on the subject of activity, producing in him a corresponding integral effect. This effect can take the form only of some integral, subject's (but not subjective) comprehension of the environment as a situation in which the present need may be satisfied, — a reflection which must be interpreted as the motivation and direction of the subject in all his subsequent activity, the set directing this behavior into the channel of reflection of the surrounding reality.

If we accept this hypothesis as a basis, we can understand that the whole of behavior, even where it has not arisen, is determined by the action of the environment, not directly, but indirectly — through the integral reflection of this environment in the subject of the activity, that is, through his sets. Individual acts of behavior and, in particular, the whole of mental activity are phenomena which are secondary in origin.

Consequently, at each given moment, of the whole of the environment, it is only that taking place in the channel of his functioning set which penetrates the mind of a subject acting in definite conditions, and is experienced by him with adequate clarity. This means that what cannot be made thinkable by attention as a formal power becomes a function of the set, and thereby becomes not only a formal, but also a purely comprehensible concept.

Hence, it becomes clear that in the conditions of impulsive behavior, the subject may have clear mental experiences despite the fact that there is no suggestion that he has exhibited attention in this case. We can see that this may take place on the basis of sets determining the subject's activity as a whole and, in particular, the working of his mind. On the basis of the set operative in each particular case, a series of mental experiences grows in the subject's consciousness and he perceives them clearly and precisely enough to guide him in his behavioral situation. Admittedly, in these conditions only those aspects or factors directly related to the current behavioral situation are experienced clearly and distinctly. For this reason, the rays of clarity and distinctness are directed toward one aspect, toward one factor of the situation, but not at the subject's will. They are dependent on the conditions in which the set acting at that particular moment was created and, perhaps, fixed. Clearly, we are here dealing only with comparatively simple situations on the basis of which a set can be created and developed satisfactorily in accordance with these conditions.

B. The Plane of Objectivization

It is a different matter when the situation necessary for solution of a problem facing a subject becomes more complex, when some obstacle arises preventing its solution. Behavior here cannot run so smooth and unobstructed a course as in the case of impulsive activity. With the appearance of an obstacle, a regular act of behavior, an individual link present in the chain of his acts, cannot usually give way rapidly to a subsequent act stimulated by it once it has arisen in man, for the obstacle actually concerns the process of this stimulation. As a result of this state of affairs, the behavior becomes held up and the link is, so to speak, wrenched out of the chain of behavioral acts. No longer giving rise to subsequent acts, for sometime it ceases to be one of the links in the chain, and psychologically it becomes an object with an independent existence, unconnected with the conditions of the current behavior, and its specific properties must first be recognized before this link can again be used purposively and once more included in the process of behavior.

Hence, with the appearance of obstacles, behavior is held up at one of its functioning links. For example, if when putting on my shoe I feel that "my foot is not properly inside the shoe," I do not completely stop my behavior directed toward putting on my shoe but merely delay it for a short time: I stop, interrupting the action of putting on my shoe. A new form of behavior then arises: The shoe, the image of which I received as a result of its perception (included in the acts of the process of putting on my shoe), since it can no longer stimulate and direct a successful and adequately purposive action of putting on my shoe, now becomes an independent object so far as I am concerned, the distinctive features of which I must recognize before I can carry on putting on my shoe, and I begin to perceive it again. The shoe becomes the object to which my perceptual acts are directed — I begin to perceive it from different aspects, assembling the features which I have noticed, trying to work out the possible reason for my failure, and also perhaps the circumstances which brought it to light. Briefly, it is on the basis of "identification" of the shoe that the process of a specially perceptual relationship to the object begins, a relationship abstracted from the interests of the immediate practical application of each of the properties which I have noted, and that the process of elementary, abstract, indirect, practical behavior is initiated.

The results of this behavior determine the subsequent course of my activity, what I must do with my shoe in order to finish purposively the process of putting it on. Clearly, I must introduce certain essential changes; I must remove the obstruction hindering the purposiveness of my behavior — in short, as a result of my abstract relationship to the object, I must carry out immediately the practical acts necessary for making my shoe ready, and only then do I resume the interrupted act of putting on my shoe.

Hence, as a result of the introduction of a complication into the situation, the process of impulsive behavior may be delayed, in which case the current link reflected primarily in the mind in the course of behavioral acts may turn into what is for me an independent object, may be excluded from the continuous chain of acts of practical behavior, and may become an object for my secondary observation, an object toward which I direct the activity of my perceptual functions in order to obtain a more detailed and clearer reflection, essential for the purposive completion of the interrupted process of my behavior.

As a result of this act, my behavior rises to a higher level — to the level of behavior motivated by perceptual acts, freed from the action of direct impulses. In these conditions, behavior is raised to the level of specifically human acts, differing qualitatively from anything that an animal might do in the ordinary conditions of its existence.

This specific act, turning an object or phenomenon included in a chain of human activity into a special, independent object of observation, may be called briefly an "act of objectivization."*

It is obvious that this act of objectivization does not create *de novo* the objects of our external environment: These objects, of course, exist independently of the subject and are the essential conditions for the development of any behavior, not necessarily belonging to that subject. They are now perceived by the subject, however, experienced as what they are, and identified. The act of objectivization implies the presence of objects in the surrounding environment to which a person might direct his acts in order to observe them repeatedly and, in this sense, to objectivate them, and finally by means of special perceptual functions, to recognize what they are.

Hence, objectivization does not create objects which exist in objective reality, independently of our actions, but turns those objects which do exist into those on which we concentrate our attention or, more strictly speaking, which we objectivate.

If we look closer into this process we may see that our behavior, included in a chain of successive acts of relationship to the environment, as it were becomes "liberated" from this chain, or "unlinked" from it, so that it becomes an independent process. A decisive role in this process of "liberation" of behavior, in its elevation to a higher, truly human level, is undoubtedly played by the act of objectivization — the act of turning a link from a chain into an independent object to which the efforts of our perceptual functions are directed. Obviously, however, this is the same act of delay, interruption, and fixation which we observe during the working of the specific state which we call "attention." Consequently, attention must be described essentially as a process of objectivization, a process in which, from the circle of our primary perceptions (that is, perceptions arising on the basis of our sets, stimulated by the

*For an experimental investigation of objectivization, see A.N. Mosiava [40, 41].

conditions of current behavioral situations), we pick out one of them which, when identified, becomes the object of our perceptual efforts and, as a result of this, becomes the clearest of all the current components of our consciousness.

Hence, the act of objectivization is a specific state characteristic of man, a state not present in animals and on which the whole superiority of man over animals is constructed — the possibility of our logical intelligence.

Special attention must be drawn to the presence of both these levels of mental life — the level of sets and the level of objectivization. Whereas the first of these levels is specific for any living being — and in particular for man in certain conditions — the second is an achievement specific to man alone, as a thinking being, laying the foundations of cultural life, the creator of cultural values.

If we examine this first level — the level of sets — we may easily see that life at this level is a continuous sequence of changes, an unending succession of the new — nothing in it is repeated, nothing is identical. Here, in the plane of the set, the main principle of existence is the principle of becoming, excluding any idea of the immutable identity of phenomena. We saw above, that reality is reflected in the mind only in those portions which are necessary for the development of a flow of activity directed toward the satisfaction of the actual needs of the living organism. This reality itself, or any of its aspects, remains entirely beyond the limits of attention of the subject, not an object for his special examination.

In the plane of sets, the outside world appears as a series of never-ending changes and continuous movement, excluding all idea of identity in an interminable series of phenomena. In short, in the plane of sets, the outside world consists of unending and unceasing change.

The second plane, giving a totally different picture of the outside world, is based on the principle of objectivization — a principle which is characteristic of this plane alone. As soon as reality begins to appear as reality, as soon as it becomes an object for man, it develops from a series of factors directly responsible for human behavior and becomes an independent object to which the subject's attention is directed, or in other words, it is objectivated.

It is on this basis that intellectual acts arise, directed toward the multilateral reflection of reality objectivated in this manner.

In contrast to reflection in the plane of sets, in the plane of objectivization we are dealing with reflection constructed on the basis of the logical principle of identity, essential for the regulation of our intellectual acts. After we have put forward an idea of one aspect of that portion of the outside world which we have objectivated, we must quickly move on to another, and then to a third, and so on, until the whole object of interest to us in this particular case is exhausted. However, when moving from one aspect to another, we shall come no closer to a satisfactory solution of the problem unless we accept that each of the aspects we examine remains before us with unchanged identity, which is necessary so that we can re-create from these images the objects as a whole: We analyze and identify each aspect of it in the course of the time necessary for completing its construction as a whole object.

Hence, the course of our mental life is changed from a living and active flow into an objectivated entity — from a segment of life it becomes the object of our thought.

II. NOTION AND IDEAS

1. Speech as an Objective Factor of the Set

We have seen that man escapes from the difficulty into which he has fallen in the increasingly complex conditions of his life by turning to the act of objectivization, to the act of an abrupt change in the direction and inner nature of his behavior. Instead of acting in a certain direction, he stops for a short time so that he can first "discuss" the situation which has arisen, and then, depending on the results of this discussion, turn again to the acts of behavior.

How does all this process take place? Do our sets play a part? These are questions which must be answered before we can form our final opinion of the character and internal structure of human activity.

In order to answer this question, our best plan is to turn to our ordinary experiments. However, a slight change is necessary, for in this case we are interested, not in the influence of the actual situation, but in the influence of a verbally created situation, acting only in the plane of ideas. The new feature which must be introduced into these experiments is that an actually perceived situation is replaced by one which is only imagined or represented verbally. Otherwise, the experiments may preserve their usual strusture.

These experiments are performed as follows: (1) Instead of giving the subject the usual fixing objects (for example, balls) we ask him to imagine that in one hand (for example, the right) he has a larger ball and in the other a smaller. As in the ordinary experiments, the fixing exposures (representations) are given repeatedly, in this case 15 times. It must be assumed that if this presentation is a factor stimulating the set, as a result of these 15 presentations the subject must fix the corresponding set. This must be found, as usual, in the critical experiments, in which the subject is shown the usual critical objects, balls of equal size.

Experiments of this type were also carried out in the optic sphere.* In this case, the experimenter proceeded as follows: Having first shown what type of stimulus had to be imagined, he asked the subject to imagine on the same screen two circles side by side, one of which had to be appreciably bigger than the other. After 15 repetitions of these presentations, the subject was shown two equal circles on the same scheme, and instructed to compare them as regards size.

The results of these experiments were as follows: Our normal illusion of the set was found in both the haptic and optic fields. Hence, a set was fixed in the subjects entirely by the action of speech; simply by imagining 15 times that balls of different sizes were acting on them, or that they saw two unequal circles, a corresponding set was fixed in these subjects — a set which subsequently prevented them for some time from adequately perceiving that objects presented to them were in fact equal.

Admittedly, illusions of this type, that is, illusions stimulated on the basis entirely of the idea of fixing objects, appeared much less frequently than illusions arising in response to the direct action of these objects, but the fact that such illusions were present is established beyond all doubt. For example, ordinary illusions of the set in the haptic sphere were found in very nearly 100% of cases, whereas here; that is, when these illusions were stimulated by verbal action, their number did not exceed 71.6%. The percentage of these illusions was lower still in the optic sphere, where the number of subjects with illusions was only 42.2% of the total.

Hence, it may be concluded from the results of these experiments that a set may also be fixed on the basis of an idea stimulated by the action of words on a subject. But it also may be concluded that this does not happen by any means so frequently as in the usual experiments. It must be assumed that, among the total number

*R. G. Natadze, "The Problem of the Fixed Set Stimulated by an Idea," Psikhologiya 1 (1942).

of subjects, a fairly high proportion of persons is found in whom a set stimulated by verbal action cannot be fixed. There is reason to suppose that these are persons characterized by the presence of some degree of anomaly – and this may be temporary and accidental, or perhaps, comparatively constant and permanent. If, however, we take a closer look at normally endowed subjects, that is, subjects with the ability to fix a set on the basis of verbal action, we must recognize that they differ considerably from one another in the degree of activity of their fixed set and in the ease of its formation. We may conclude from the results of our experiments that whereas a large number of normal subjects can fix a set on the basis of verbal action only to a very weak degree, a comparatively small number of subjects, consisting mainly of actors and students of drama, are unusually well endowed in this respect. They can fix a set on the basis of an idea in almost 100% of cases, and moreover, they can fix it strongly.*

1. If we examine sets fixed in this way from the point of view of their stability, we note that a set, stimulated by verbal action, generally shows a comparatively low degree of stability. Of 16 subjects in whom a set was fixed in these conditions, in 15 (93.8%) comparatively slight fixation of the set was found, and only one subject exhibited a set which could be regarded as strongly fixed.

Hence, fixation of the set by this method is distinguished by the much lower degree of stability than is found after fixation of a set by the action of an actual situation.

2. The comparatively low degree of fixation of a set fixed on the basis of an idea is also reflected in its other aspects, especially the degree of its stability and its excitability. These experiments clearly showed that, during testing of the stability of a fixed set of the type in which we are interested (tests were made on 13 subjects giving a well-defined picture of fixation of a verbally stimulated set), at the end of intervals of 5 to 15 minutes after the fixation experiment, the set persisted in 5 subjects (38.4%) of the total; moreover, apart from one subject in whom the phenomenon of a static set was observed, all these subjects showed a very weak degree of fixation. Two of them gave two illusions each, and two gave one illusion each.

Hence, in these experiments the degree of stability of the fixed set was very low. These results show that a verbally stimulating

*R. G. Natadze, op. cit.

set is, in general, much less stable than the set arising as a result of the direct action of the actual situation.

3. The same may be said concerning the excitability of this type of set. As a result of 5 fixing exposures in the haptic sphere, a set could be fixed in only 7 of 13 subjects in whom the general set could be verbally stimulated. If we compare this number with the number of subjects with excitability of the set in response to actual stimulation it is unquestionably very low. First, the lower threshold of excitability is much higher (whereas in that case one exposure is sufficient in order to produce a noticeable effect of fixation, in this case for the same purpose 5 fixing exposures are necessary). Second, whereas in the usual experiments the number of persons with such a threshold is comparatively high, in this case it is not more than 23%. Third, this illusion is very weak, for in one subject it persisted until the third exposure, in another until the second, and in the third only during the first exposure.

Hence, we see that a verbally stimulated set is much more difficult to evoke than the ordinary fixed set.

4. Does the process of extinction of this set show any special features? Examination of the results of this investigation shows the following points:

A. Of the 36 subjects showing the effect of fixation of the set, 9 (25%) were subjects with a static type of set. They gave an illusion of contrast which remained unchanged for more than 30 exposures. In the ordinary experiments with normal persons, this did not happen, and there were not more than 3 to 5% of subjects with such static sets. Further experiments must show the basis on which this distinguishing feature of the verbally fixed set lies.

B. In a particularly high proportion (52%) of subjects, a coarse dynamic set is detected. These are people who gave an illusion of contrast from the very beginning and maintained it without appreciable change until they finally observed that the critical objects were equal.

C. Finally, in 25% of all subjects a plastic set is found; this number also is not high compared to sets based on actual situations rather than on imaginary ones.

All these differences in the process of extinction of a verbally fixed set were obtained in R. G. Natadze's earliest experiments, carried out to study the possibility of the existence of this type of set. Further experiments must show what must be preserved from these results and what must be changed in one way or another.

2. The Problem of the "Idea"

If we survey all that we have obtained as a result of these experiments, we must recognize that fixation of the set on the basis of verbal action undoubtedly occurs. Speech is a specific sphere of reality for us, on the basis of which man has built a new stratum of sets, responsible for and controlling his behavior.

The problem which now faces us may be expressed as follows: How does it come about that speech begins to play in this case the same role as objective reality, on the basis of which our activity usually develops? Certainly it is not our external environment, the situation currently acting upon us, which is the factor directly determining the appearance of the set, but merely a verbally reflected form of that environment. We could say that the objective factor responsible for the origin of the set in this case is not an actual situation but merely a verbally stimulated situation. This means that the type of set which arises here in the subject depends not on the conditions in which he has to act, but on the type of reality that he reflects in his expressions, that he wishes to express with his speech.

Hence, whereas in our ordinary experiments with sets we always had to deal with some individual fragment of reality, with a definite situation for the particular person concerned, in this case the objective condition for the development of the set is merely an imaginary situation, based on ideas; the subject has to contend not with a real fact, but merely with an imaginary situation represented by ideas.

The objected conditions of formation of the set differ significantly from each other in these two cases. Whereas in ordinary cases of action of the set the objective situation is relatively real, in this case the situation does not in fact exist but is merely imagined. Hence, we must recognize that in these conditions a completely new stratum of sets is concerned, a new stratum which can be found only in subjects working with ideas, notions, or thoughts.

What exactly is this idea? It might be supposed that it is the usual notion, "the reproduced image of an object based on our past experience." In the experiments mentioned above, however, we obtained results which did not justify the drawing of this conclusion. Ideas of the same object or phenomenon, as we know, may differ from each other, first in the degree of their intensity or brightness. However, these experiments show that the factor of intensity or brightness is unimportant: Ideas may be of maximal brightness, yet incapable of stimulating the activity of the subject. Consequently, we must recognize that it is not the representation, the simple form of an object that plays the decisive role in these cases, but something completely different.

3. The "Idea" in Dreams

In order to obtain a clearer picture of the nature of the specific processes lying at the basis of the subject's behavior in these cases, we must analyze a series of observations in which not only human subjects but also animals appear to have experiences similar to those with which we are now concerned. These are dreams, which evidently are found even among people in the most primitive stages of development, in children in the earliest periods of their life, and also in animals.

We must recognize, of course, that dreams are not experiences with an active meaning. Nevertheless, they are witnessed facts even at primitive stages of development, where there is evidently no such thing as true intellectual activity.

One observation will suffice. A hunting dog lies beside me and sleeps. According to all the signs it is not resting; it whimpers, from time to time it barks, although admittedly quietly, yet clearly enough to show that in this case it is the normal bark which it uses specifically when pursuing game. Everything points to the fact that the dog is "dreaming" a hunting scene in which it seems to be taking part.

There is no need to discuss children's dreams: They are so common that they give rise to no doubts. The same must be said concerning the dreams of primitive man. Facts of this type are well established and we need have no hesitation in making use of them.

But if this is so, if there is no doubt about dreams at these comparatively primitive stages of development, this means that we must accept that the possibility of ideas is equally well established at these stages of development. The animal, in this case the dog, has definite images and they evoke corresponding reactions — the dog begins to bark. The same may be said regarding human dreams; there can be no doubt about the presence of ideas in them. The whole content of dreams in general is built up from images of ideas.

Attention must be drawn, however, to one special aspect of dreams. If we examine carefully these "ideas" in dreams, we see that they are constantly being transformed, and as soon as they appear they are turned into perception. This happens so often that we may doubt whether in a state of dreaming in general, we may have any ideas whatever, in the true meaning of the word. Once the doubts about the presence of the process of modification of our "ideas" into images of perception have been cleared up, there can likewise be no doubt about the existence of the idea. However, this entity is often distinctive and so specific in character that it becomes difficult to regard it as ordinary or genuine. The images of our ideas during sleep, as we have just mentioned, as soon as our attention is turned to them begin to change into images of perception. What originally begins to appear in consciousness simply as a series of separate ideas is quickly transformed into actual experiences, genuine perception, into phenomenon which actually begin to unfold before our eyes. The thoughts which enter the mind during sleep are at once given a concrete form and begin to be experienced as genuine, actual perception. This transformation is experienced so clearly that there can be no doubt about it, no doubt that if we think of something during sleep, we see that the images of this reminiscence soon begin to pass before our eyes as genuine, clear phenomena of perception.

This observation gives a particularly accurate definition of what takes place in our consciousness during dreams. In sleep, everything that we imagine is quickly transformed into images of perception.

This undoubted fact that ideas are turned into images of perception is of considerable interest from the points of view of the problem of the psychological features of dreams. If this type of transformation of images of ideas into images of perception is possible, it can be deduced that they are indistinguishable from each other in meaning in dreams: If perception is the reflection of concrete reality, the reflection of a particular situation as it affects an individual, the same must also be said regarding ideas during sleep; otherwise, their transformation into perception would be completely impossible. If a particular image can be immaterially the image of an idea or of perception, this means that these are indistinguishable, and that the same image can serve for both in each individual case. This means that perception and idea in a dream state cannot be differentiated; they are diffuse experiences, and ideas are just as concrete and individual in their content as is perception. Consequently, the statement that the content of ideas is to some extent generalized in character in this case rests on an insecure basis.

Admittedly, where the content is indefinite or diffuse, it becomes difficult to identify it accurately as an experience of ideation or perception. However, the facts of our consciousness do not become generalized because of this: In this case they are simply diffuse and indeterminate in character, but they do not cease to be an experience — admittedly indeterminate, but nevertheless with a perfectly individual content.

In similar cases we have, in principle, not a generalized content, not an aggregate of general signs of some group of phenomena or objects, but simply an indeterminate, diffuse experience which, because of this diffuseness, is difficult or impossible to place in a category of a particular individual content.

Hence, we may conclude that the ideas which we have in a dream state are indistinguishable from perception in the basic properties of their content — they change from one to the other without any change in content: In a dream state as a general rule, differentiation of ideas and perceptions does not occur.

4. Ideas Based on Verbal Action

If by ideas we mean experiences which usually form the content of dreams, we must assume that they do not differ in principle from perception and that they may take place, not only in man at different stages of development, but also in animals.

Hence, we see that the ideas lying at the basis of the experiments with sets formed in response to verbal stimulation must not be identified with "ideas" in the narrow meaning of this word. These latter may take place at comparatively early stages of development — not only in dreams — whereas the ideas stimulated on the basis of verbal action may be detected only in the living being possessing the power of speech — in man.

The fact that in this case we are not concerned with individual ideas is clear from the role of speech. Speech never directly expresses any form of concrete, individual image. It always generalizes, it always applies to some more or less general meaning. Rather, then, we must assume that in this case we are concerned with a more generalized process than in the case of an idea. We have reason to suppose that we are digressing here from the concrete sphere of what is only perceived or only imagined, and we are climbing to the higher sphere of what is thought.

This means that in these cases the specifically human feature formed at the highest degrees of its development comes into its own right — intellectual activity begins.

It thus becomes clear that in man a second, and higher form of set appears, characterized above all by the fact that, besides the need which stimulates its activity, it requires also the presence of a situation definable in the categories of thought and not of perception, as is the case of a set operating on the actual plane.

The following situation is obtained: Man has developed the ability to act in a new plane, the plane of secondary reflection of reality, and he is thus able not only to respond directly to stimuli acting upon him, which is also to some degree possible for animals, but also to react indirectly in various ways to the wider picture of reality unfolding before his eyes.

5. Experiments on the Basis of Representations and Ideas

A curious phenomenon was discovered in one of R. G. Natadze's investigations, which he described as follows: "The psychological nature of scenic re-creation lies in the formation of a set corresponding to the situation imagined (but not perceived) at a particular moment; the set evoked by the idea is fixed in the process of repetition" [45]. Natadze concludes that it is far easier to fix a set in a talented actor by means of an idea than in persons unconnected with the stage or with little ability to act. Characteristically, the ability to fix sets on the basis of ideas is much more highly developed in gifted drama students than in those with fewer talents. Natadze shows by a wide range of experiments that his conclusion is well grounded; it is justified in the most varied combinations of experimental conditions.

In order to demonstrate the considerable difference in this respect between highly talented actors and those less talented, we may turn to the results shown in Table XVI. This table shows that the more talented actors gave results very different from persons unconnected with the stage. The difference in this case was considerable; although the possibility is not ruled out that among the subjects, selected at random, who had no connection with the theater, there may have been some who were capable actors, their results (31.1%) were nevertheless less than half those obtained by the professional actors (87.8%) and the capable drama students (80%). Clearly, therefore, artistic talent shows a high degree of positive

TABLE XVI

	Number of subjects	Adequate responses (%)	Illusion (%)	Weak illusion (%)	Average (%)	Strong (%)	Continuous illusion (%)
Experienced actors	10	10	90	22.2	33.3	33.3	11.1
Young actors	7	14.3	85.27	33.3	33.3	33.3	--
Capable drama students	10	20	80	25	25	37.5	12.5
Persons with no connection with the stage	25	69.8	30.1	75	8.3	8.3	8.3

correlation with the number of illusions of sets stimulated by the subject's imagination (in these experiments, the subject was instructed verbally to imagine that in his right hand he had a large ball and in his left a smaller ball). A particularly interesting feature is that these results were not substantially changed when the experimental conditions were made more complicated, as, for example, when the subjects were allowed to see actual stimuli completely opposite to the imaginary fixing objects.

Charpentier's objects, equal in weight but different in volume, were placed in the subject's hands. Consequently, nothing prevented him from receiving the corresponding illusion. However, the subject was instructed to imagine that the weights were distributed in the opposite direction to their actual order, and consequently to imagine that the lighter object was on the side which felt heavier, and the heavier object was on the side which felt lighter.

The results of these experiments show that, by means of imagination, subjects can overcome the strength of the action of Charpentier's illusion. Whereas in these conditions persons unconnected with the stage (moderately skilled workmen) had no illusions whatever, among the subjects who were talented actors their number reached 65.2%. This figure clearly demonstrates the great difference between these categories of subjects.

It may be concluded that the incidence of illusions of the set in these conditions shows a high degree of positive correlation with dramatic talent.

The results of this variant of the experiment also show that sets can be fixed on the basis of ideas even when the idea is obviously contrary to the actual perception in the same modality. If, for example, a subject has in his hands objects of the same volume, in suitable conditions the set may be fixed in this subject that in his right hand he has a larger object than in his left hand. Moreover, this happens much more often (77.8%) in talented actors than in ordinary subjects chosen at random in relation to this qualification (23.8%).

Without dwelling on the other variants of these experiments, we can reach the general conclusion that ability to fix a set on the basis of the idea of an object, when opposite to what is actually perceived, is far more widespread among talented actors than among persons with no connection with the stage, and also than students of drama who, as shown by reports on their work, display little artistic ability.

To sum up, we may conclude from various experiments that a fixed set on the basis of an idea may be formed far more frequently in talented artists than in persons lacking in such talent.

What do these results show us? We mentioned above that in these and in other further experiments it is not the capacity for vivid imagination — the imagination of dreamlike diffuse experience — but rather the capacity for an idea or thought in general that is investigated. However, the results of the experiments with talented actors evidently disagree fundamentally with this suggestion. We have no reason to suppose that such actors surpass our ordinary subjects in their ability to think. There are other ways in which we may obtain reliable information to judge the intellectual powers of our subjects, and their results do not always coincide with the results of these experiments. This fact compels us to ask: What do our experiments really investigate — thoughts, ideas, or simply the capacity for imagining individual events?

To solve this problem we studied some of the results obtained during these experiments. First, we examined the great difference between the two categories of subjects. Whereas the talented actors easily solved the problem of imagining the solution in a sense opposite to the actual facts, subjects having no connection with the stage in most cases either solved the problem with considerable difficulty or failed completely to do so. Most subjects of this second group felt themselves to be under an excessive strain during the solution: "I must collect all my strength" ... "the strain is quite unusual" ... "you know, this has made me very tired" ... "I am absolutely worn out..." were the remarks made by the subjects of this category. If, eventually, they succeeded in solving the problem, it was only after a long series of attempts; sometimes 15 to 26 exposures were necessary before the subjects of this category could carry out the task given to them, whereas 3 to 5 exposures were enough for the talented actors.

Briefly, the results show that whereas talented artists easily solve problems of this type, ordinary subjects are comparatively unable to do so.

It is very important to note how this process takes place in persons solving the problem comparatively easily. When the problem was made more complicated by special experimental conditions, the subject noticed difficulty in solving it. These cases are particularly interesting for defining the method of solution used by the subjects of this category — the talented actors.

The subject fixes the idea required by the problem, but suddenly and unexpectedly it is lost, and for a short time the subject stops, having nothing to bring the necessary idea to life again: "It has disappeared again" . . . "it has come back again!" said one actress. "I found it, but it slipped away again! How difficult this seems!" said another subject.

Hence, we see that, despite a considerable increase in the complexity of the experimental conditions, generally speaking the subjects of this category solved the problem relatively easily, and much more easily than persons unconnected with the stage.

From these results we may determine the nature of the difference between the behavior of these two groups of subjects. One group — the talented actors — tune themselves comparatively easily to the solution of the problem — they easily activate in themselves what is required — 3 to 5 exposures are enough to evoke the required image, easily produce the idea required of them. On the other hand, the method of formation of this idea in these subjects is specific; it is "switched on" or "switched off" . . . they either "have" it or they "have not." The impression is gained that this idea is either present, ready made, or is absent until it suddenly makes it appearance.

These findings give a clear indication of the nature of these "ideas." They must be assumed to be mental acts, differing significantly from whatever it is that controls the behavior of the subjects unconnected with the theater in these experiments. Whereas the latter mostly use acts of thought or ideas, as we prefer to call them, in their behavior, the talented actors, when faced with the solution of these problems, as a rule do not use acts of thought but vivid, individual images, imagination of definite events, which arise and act as integral images either present in consciousness as fully completed entities or completely absent from consciousness, experiences analogous to the undifferentiated scenes enacted in our dreams. In this way they differ radically from what was found in these cases in our ordinary subjects who had no specific dramatic talents. We might sum up in a few words the difference between them: Whereas in talented actors in the situation of our experiments, definite individual images or vivid undifferentiated scenes appear, other subjects, in the same conditions, develop ideas or thoughts which begin to determine their activity through corresponding forms of sets.

There is, of course, no doubt whatever about the ability of our first group of subjects to "think," that in suitable conditions they may demonstrate this ability; but in the present case the experimental conditions are such that they stimulate the activity of their figurative imagination rather than their general processes of thought. If, on the other hand, with the other group of subjects this does not happen, if some form of abstract thought rather than the ability of concrete imagination is activated in this group, then it must be assumed that this takes place simply because figurative imagination in these subjects does not exist to the degree in which it is found in the first category.

Hence, the results of experiments to stimulate sets on the basis of ideas show that, whereas in talented actors, individual concrete images of "scenes" are produced, in ordinary subjects comparatively more generalized mental experiences are formed.

III. THOUGHT AND WILL

1. Thought Takes Place on the Basis of Objectivization

We know that ideas which may be found in animals, are much more common in man. The characteristic feature of this mental act is that above all it is direct; that is, in the subject's own experience it is never opposed to the act of perception. Both idea and perception are experienced as qualities of an object. Whether these properties are actual or not is not fully considered here, as it is, for example, in a dream state, when experience, perception, and ideas arise on the basis of an actual set.

We have seen above that at the human stage of development the subject is rarely confronted with an insuperable obstacle. When he is, however, his behavior becomes incapable of further development and the subject is forced to stop and to give up his impulsive behavior. But, whereas in similar cases an animal in fact does stop his present behavior in order to change to a new type, the same cannot be said with respect to man — he does not stop his present behavior because he decides finally to give it up: He decides to stop these acts simply because he hopes by so doing to continue them later more successfully. This cessation of his behavioral acts by no means implies the complete abandonment of all activity by the subject. Far from it! As we have seen above, a new and distinctive stratum of activity is present in man, as a result of which the activity may be successfully continued. At this stage of behavior, the repeated experience or, more accurately, the objectivization of the developing obstacle takes place. Interruption of current behavior and the cessation of its activity are necessary in order that this repeated experience may be obtained.

Hence, we see that the act of objectivization arrests the flow of behavior and in its place substitutes conditions enabling repeated experience and, consequently, the trial and study of the conditions of behavior on this basis.

How is this act carried out? How can man study his objectivated behavior and what are his opportunities for doing so?

When, in the process of our behavior, conditions arise compelling us to turn to acts of objectivization, the following questions arise: "What has happened?" "Why has this happened?" "What would have happened if things had been different?" These questions call for immediate solution.

It cannot be otherwise! In the process of development of behavior I meet with a difficulty which cannot be quickly and directly removed, and for this reason, it evokes in me the need to explain, in the first place, the character of this difficulty, and the possibility of its removal.

In this case, just as in the case of development of ordinary impulsive behavior, the subject develops a need which strives to obtain satisfaction. The position is just the same as in every case of ordinary behavior — a need and a situation for its satisfaction — these are the two conditions necessary for the appearance of a particular act of behavior.

But at the same time, there is an obvious difference between these two cases. The need arising on the basis of objectivization has a perfectly definite character — it is a problem which must be solved in the plane of perceptual or, we may say, theoretical, but not practical activity, as in the case of impulsive activity. It stands outside the limits of actual practical problems, it is above these limits, and it cannot therefore serve its interests directly. It tries rather to shed light on circumstances, it is more a theoretical than a practical problem, which is usually solved in the primary plane of reflection of reality.

In any act of human behavior we see the following picture: A subject performs a more or less complex act of behavior when a large obstacle blocks the way to further activity. In such a case he feels compelled to interrupt his activity, to stop; and, instead of performing the next act of behavior, he turns to objectivization. This enables him to transfer the activity of his behavior to a theoretical region — he turns to thought in order to solve the problem confronting him, and thus to satisfy the specific need arising on the basis of objectivization.

Human thought arises in this way. It is a mental activity set in motion only on the basis of objectivization and directed toward the satisfaction of a theoretical, perceptual need, stimulated in this manner. Consequently, it is clear that thought, in the true meaning of the word, is only possible if objectivization is possible, and that in a sphere of activity where there is no objectivization, there can be no true thought. Hence, thought, in the true meaning of the word, appears only at the human level of mental development, so that all the attempts of bourgeois psychologists to identify the presence of thought processes at the levels of mental development of animals seem to me to be fruitless and unscientific.

Objectivization, like thought which arises on its basis, is a subtlety which is completely foreign to the first plane of behavior, but absolutely essential for its second plane.

However, it would be wrong to think that the faculty of objectivization alone is sufficient for thought activity. The participation here of the set is just as necessary as in the first plane of activity. What part do we attribute to the set in the presence of thought processes? What special features are found in these conditions?

Suppose I turn to an act of habitual behavior, for example, I pick up a pen and start to write. I soon note, however, that from time to time I write badly, in places my handwriting becomes indistinct. I have therefore to keep examining what I have written in order to correct it. I soon stop writing and try to find the reason for my slowness — I want to know what is preventing me from writing — is it the pen which I must change or perhaps is there some other reason? On the basis of a particular set, I set in motion the corresponding activity — I begin to write. Soon, however, I find that something restrains me — my activity is slowed down a little. This compels me to stop my activity and to turn to an act of objectivization. On the basis of this act, instead of continuing my activity, I begin to consider what is stopping me from writing. In brief, on the basis of objectivization, I begin to carry out acts of thought in order to discover how I should alter my behavior to make it more productive. The process of thought in this case also cannot take place completely independently of the subject's sets. Eact act of judgment undoubtedly arises from the corresponding set, and the problem is to determine what this set is in each individual case, and whence it comes.

In the first place it must be noted that in this case we have a set arising, not on the basis of an actual need and corresponding situation, but on the basis of a secondary, an imaginary need and its situation. In each individual case the subject is confronted with a problem (a need for cognition) and the idea of a situation for its satisfaction, as a result of which a definite set appears. Subsequently, each individual, independent act of thought arises on the basis of this set, and consequently, represents an individual case of its realization.

In the present case, for example, a set is produced, constructed on the basis of objectivated material — man's logical thought arises and takes place in the same way.

We have already considered above attempts to analyze some of these main conditions of this thought. As we know, our thought requires the presence of a certain number of established and indispensable conditions. The first of these, of course, is the presence of what are called the fundamental axiomatic laws of thought. For our purpose, however, it will be sufficient to examine only one of these — the law of identity as the principal and most typical of all the laws of thought.

The principal axiomatic law of logical thought is the law that everything is equal to itself, that A = A.

What does this law tell us? Evidently that if we abstract something from the unceasing world movement and re-experience it, we see that everything equals itself, that A = A. Otherwise, if

A were placed opposite to A, that is, if some phenomenon or other were compared with itself, it would be necessary to re-examine it and to re-experience it as the same thing — once in the role of subject and again in the role of predicate.

The fact that an essential condition of logical thought is the axiomatic law of identity shows that logical thought deals with reality as such, that is, with re-experienced reality, with reality as an object, but not as a constantly changing course.

It thus becomes clear that an essential basis of our logical thought is the fact of objectivization, on the foundations of which is created the ability to experience identity, that logical thought is possible only at the stage of development at which the presence of objectivization is an established fact, and that this thought consequently is found only at the human level of development.

2. The Will as Another, Specifically Human, Function

Thought is used to solve a theoretical problem facing us in the conditions of objectivated reality. Ultimately, however, this problem serves all the interests of practical life. However far a theoretical problem may go, it ultimately, directly or indirectly, is concerned with problems of human practical activity. The need for objectivization always and only arises when circumstances become more complicated — when difficulties arise in the solution of problems, and acts of thought become necessary only in these cases.

But as soon as a series of problems or an individual problem is solved, a new task then arises — the task of the practical application of the intellectually solved problem. Expressed in another way, a subject faced with a practical problem turns to an act of behavior which would guarantee for him the full practical application of his theoretically obtained results. Henceforward, the problem is concerned with ability to switch from the plane of objectivization to the plane of actual behavior. The subject is faced with the problem of applying practically what he recognized theoretically to be worthwhile — the problem of performing corresponding volitional acts.

How is this done?

The problem in this case is essentially the ability to put into action a set corresponding to an act of behavior that has become necessary. The appearance of such a set is sufficient to ensure the performance of this act. The purpose of the volitional act, consequently, is precisely this, that is, turning a set created in the plane of objectivization into an actual set — into a force directing human activity into a definite direction.

IV. CONCLUSIONS

When an animal repeats the same activity, this is essentially not a true repetition. The animal in each individual case performs a new act of behavior — it does not experience it as the same act. This means that repetition, as such, does not exist for an animal.

It is a different matter with man. When man encounters difficulty in performing a certain act, he pauses in his action and concentrates on one of the factors, which he considers to be at the center of the difficulty — he objectivates this factor, and dwells on it consciously for some time. Consequently, he picks it out from the current process of behavior, isolates it, and turns it into the object of a new type of behavior — intellectual behavior.

The animal, also, may dwell on one of the factors of its behavior, but this is not a real interruption in behavior, because to the animal, which has no awareness of identity, this is not the same factor. The situation is different with man. He may perform acts of objectivization, and on this basis he may develop consciousness of identity.

But what is the fundamental difference between the mind of animals and man? It is based on the cardinal difference existing between animals and man — the fact that man is a social being. Man lives and acts, that is, exists, not only for himself, but also for others. As a social being, his life crosses the frontiers of his own existence and becomes, in fact, a part of reality for another: We must be particularly careful to contrast "society," as an "abstraction," with the individual. The individual is a social being. For this reason, the manifestation of his life is the manifestation and personification of social life.* Consciousness of objective existence must undoubtedly be formed in the life of man, the social being, at the same time as his social qualities are formed. Power of objectivization could only be developed on the basis of social attributes, so that this power clearly forms a specific feature of the human mind.

What were the changes which must have brought this about?

In the first place, the human mind must have developed its

*Marx and Engels, Works, Vol. 3, p. 624.

activity on the basis of objectivization. We have seen that this actually happened and that man became possessed of the power of speech, a thinking being. His intellectual functions appeared and became his guiding force.

Next, along with and on the basis of this objectivization, in the field of human activity a new change was found, one which was undoubtedly of fundamental importance. Man developed a will, or the ability to direct his behavior freely, by following the indications of his intellect.

Hence, both intellect and will are formed on the basis of objectivization. However, the possibility is not ruled out that both perception and memory have also developed a relationship with it, and as a result of this, have become definitely active processes. However, for this to happen, the participation of thought must be added to the activity of these functions, for thought can give these intrinsically passive processes a definitely active character. In this case, the place of this type of passive perception is occupied by observation, and the place of the no less passive reproduction by active recollection.

These are the changes found in the mind of man as a social being.

According to this description, it is easy to see that the traditional classification of mental processes into perceptual, emotional, and volitional does not at all correspond to the objectivate state of affairs. The mind should rather be considered from the point of view of development, in which case the fallacy of the position of traditional bourgeois psychology in the analysis of mental processes would become clear.

But if this is true, in this case we must distinguish two levels of mental activity — the level of sets, at which, besides affective, we should find undifferentiated perceptual and reproductive elements, and the level of objectivization, at which we should find definitely active forms of mental activity — thought and will.

The level of sets has been identified in the ordinary phenomena of acts of everyday behavior. The level of objectivization is quite a different matter. We have risen to its level only when we are confronted with a new and difficult problem demanding a correspondingly new solution. In this case, we have first to turn to the acts of objectivization and then, on its basis, to thought processes, giving us essential aid in finding the set whose realization rests on our will.

Such are the unique features of human psychology, distinguishing it radically from the psychology of the animal.

V. INDIVIDUAL TYPES OF SET

The aspects of the activity of the set, described above, unquestionably demand more detailed investigations which, it is hoped, would not only clarify the differential-psychological concepts established above, but would also reveal new concepts which would perhaps be no less productive in developing our knowledge of the set than those mentioned above. The need for further research in this direction is urgent.

However, the differential-psychological aspect of the theory of sets is not the only factor which we must consider at this point. There are many more questions to which we can give more or less satisfactory answers. I have in mind not the special differential-psychological questions such as we have considered so far, but problems of a more general class — problems of the typological value of our concept of the set, and problems of the types of sets in different individuals.

We will first consider whether the various aspects of sets which we have discovered are merely accidental variations or whether they are distinct factors of a unified structure, finding its expression in the specific combination of individual aspects of sets of the personality.

As a result of many years of study of phenomena in this category, I have accumulated extensive material which provides a conclusive answer to this question. It is true that specific combinations of individual aspects are found, which, together with the faculty of objectivization, characterize the sets of a particular subject as ideas of a definite type.

This question is undoubtedly extremely important. The set is the fundamental factor in human activity, the factor on which this activity grows, and if we find that certain definite types of activity of sets exist, which appear dependent on the individual characteristics of the subject of this activity, we shall then have to recognize that sets possess something akin to typologically different forms of manifestation, and that, consequently, it is necessary to make a special study of these forms.

1. Sets of Different Types of People

How can we solve this problem? It is evidently fairly easy. We must choose a large enough number of people differing typologically from one another to a considerable degree, and, as a result of observation of them, we must divide them into several groups and then investigate the fixed sets of these groups. It must be remembered that the sets of the subjects of these groups are studied in all their differential-psychological manifestations. The results obtained enable us to define clearly enough the sets of each of these groups, so that we can then describe the subjects from the point of view of differences in their fixed sets.

Adequate facts of this nature are available, and on their basis we have attempted to solve this problem [61]. We have found that from the point of view of differences of their fixed sets, human beings can be divided into three main groups. Without going into the question of subgroups, we may describe the first group as composed of persons with a dynamic set or, simply, as a group of dynamic persons, the second as a group of static persons, and, finally, the third as a group of variable persons. Let us examine each of these groups.

A. Dynamic Persons

Experiments to investigate sets were carried out in the usual manner. Let us assume that these experiments in all cases concerned three sensory modalities — optic, haptic, and muscular. The fixability of sets was studied in each of these sensory spheres separately, at first in one group (the most numerous) and later in the other groups consisting of smaller numbers. In the case of the first group of subjects, that is, the group of dynamic persons, we found similar pictures of the state of the fixed set in all three sensory modalities investigated. This result may be regarded as one of the specific properties inherent in persons of this category. In particular, so far as the state of excitability of fixation of the set is concerned, persons of this group reached their optimum of illusion in all three sensory modalities after 15 fixing exposures. With an increase or decrease in this number, the number of illusions began to fall. Naturally, not all the sensory modalities tested gave exactly the same number of illusions, but the variations in these cases were so slight that they may be disregarded, and we may conclude that the excitability of the fixed set of the category of subjects with which we are concerned was identical.

And so, the excitability of the fixed set in subjects belonging to the same group is basically similar in pattern. This excitability is not very high, but neither is it very low.

However, there are some persons standing very close to this main group, but very slightly differing from it typologically, in whom the excitability is either much higher than the excitability of sets in the main category of our subjects or, conversely, much below it. Our main category of subjects occupies a middle place in this respect: Whereas the optimum of excitability of sets in these subjects amounted to 15, in others the number was 2 in one case and 25 to 30 in the other.

We must next consider the types of course of the fixed set in this group of subjects. On analyzing the appropriate data, we found, as might have been expected, that in this group of subjects the predominant type was one of a plastic and dynamic fixed set (on the average 83% in all three sensory modalities studied). The remaining types were represented in this group in such small numbers that they may be disregarded. It must be noted, however, that this same group of subjects also included persons with a coarse dynamic set. It thus appeared that the great majority of our subjects were characterized by the dynamic nature of their sets, so that a suitable name for the persons of this category would be the group of "dynamic persons."

Let us now turn to the question of the rigidity of this type of set in our subjects. Experimental results showed that the mean numbers for all subjects varied between the following limits: The mean coefficient in the optic sphere was 13.5, in the haptic 15.7, and in the muscular 11.4. This means that, despite the slight difference in the number of the results, on the whole it is reasonable to conclude that the fixed set in our subjects was fairly stable.

The degree of constancy of the fixed set is shown by the following figures: in the optic sphere 87.8%, in the haptic 78.8%, and in the muscular 87.8%. These figures are high enough to indicate that the fixed set of the category of persons whom we studied is as a rule fairly constant.

At the same time, it is also highly stable. In the optic modality, 84.8% of our subjects (33 in all) showed a stable form of set for several days (5 series of experiments), in the haptic sphere nearly 100%, and, finally, in the muscular sphere 87.8%.

Data concerning the degree of irradiation of the set were as follows:

(a). In experiments with irradiation from the optic to the haptic sphere, irradiation was found in 75% of our subjects, although it should be noted that the irradiated set in these cases was weak, as expressed by the comparatively high coefficient of cases of assimilative illusions, which are known to occur mainly in the presence of weak fixation.

(b). The percentage of irradiation in the opposite direction was somewhat lower; a set fixed in the haptic region irradiated to the optic region in only 67% of our cases; here, also, it was weak, although not so weak as in cases of irradiation in the opposite direction, that is, in the case of irradiation from the optic to the haptic region.

(c). Cases of irradiation from the optic region to the muscular were found almost as often (66.3%). In some of the subtypes of this group of subjects, however, these cases reached high values (up to 100%). Finally, irradiation in the opposite direction, that is, from the muscular modality to the optic, was found in only 62% of our subjects. As might have been expected, irradiation took place particularly easily in subjects who showed it to the maximal degree in experiments in the opposite direction.

Hence, it is clear that the subjects of the type at present being studied were characterized by irradiation of sets from one sensory modality to another — irradiation which is fairly extensive, but which in most cases remains comparatively low in intensity.

If we seek a general description of the fixed set in persons whom we describe as dynamic, we may summarize our results on this problem as follows: The optimum of excitability of the fixed set of these persons varies from 10 to 15 fixing exposures; their sets are dynamic in type, they are constant, rigid within average limits, and they are capable of irradiation and are intermodally stable.

Other variants of the subjects of this type are also found, but there is no need to discuss them specially here, for they are comparatively few in number and differ only very slightly from the representatives of our main type. The indices of optimal excitability of sets and of their stability and irradiation are slightly lower in these persons than in the representatives of our main type, but otherwise they resemble them completely.

Hence, it is clear that on the whole, persons of this type resemble each other sufficiently closely in the individual aspects and forms of their fixed sets that they can be regarded as representatives of one definite type of set.

Special observations have shown that the persons of this typological group possess a well-developed power of objectivization. As soon as the need for putting this power into operation arises, it is transformed into an active state. Attention should be paid here to the specific properties of the objectivization of these dynamic subjects, to the ease with which it is put into action, and the smoothness of its course. In these cases we do not at all have the impression that acts of objectivization encounter any considerable obstacles which must be overcome before they may be put into operation. As we shall see below, this occurs in our static subjects, who frequently experience a pathological internal struggle before they can secure their objectivated goals.

Hence, a well-developed power of objectivization and the ability to change over easily toward objectivated purposes are features which should be stressed, particularly when defining persons with dynamic sets.

Besides persons with sets having dynamic structure, who constitute the great majority of human beings, the healthy members of society, there are others with sets slightly different from this normal form. Most of these are persons with static sets. In most cases, these are energetic members of society, successfully coping with their problems. They frequently attract attention by their untiring activity at work, but nevertheless they differ considerably from the ordinary healthy members of society and their life and activity assume certain specific features. It is interesting to examine the forms taken by the fixed sets of these individuals.

B. Static Persons

1. So far as the problem of the speed of fixation of sets or their excitability is concerned, we find that in the majority of persons in this category the figure is fairly high: 88% of subjects fixed their sets after only 2 presentations of the experimental objects; in this case however, the set which develops is admittedly coarse, but it is still dynamic in form. If the number of fixing exposures is increased to 5 or 10, the dynamic sets give way to a static form, and the results obtained with most of these subjects show that this is the optimal number of fixing exposures. Hence, we may conclude that the optimal excitability of the fixed set in persons of this category is 5 to 10 exposures.

2. What forms of sets are predominant in the subjects of this category? The results of experiments in different sensory modalities show that the characteristic form of set in persons of this category is a coarse, static, fixed set. It is this form of set most frequently found in the subjects investigated (89 to 100%). This group of subjects is therefore described as a group of "static" persons, as opposed to dynamic.

3. Constancy of the sets was found in almost 100% of cases (from 90 to 100%). The same was true of its stability (100%). In nearly all these cases (90%), the sets preserved their coarse, static character.

4. At the same time, it was found that the fixed sets of this group of subjects irradiate extensively. They spread from the optic region to the haptic and muscular region, and from the latter back to the optic and haptic regions.

The same is true of the haptic set, which passes without hindrance to the other two sensory regions. In nearly all cases, the irradiating set remains coarse and static in form. Characteristically, in the great majority of cases the illusions were illusions of contrast, and this form remained dominant in almost every case of irradiation of the set.

Hence, we may conclude that the fixed sets of static persons are highly excitable, coarse, static, intermodal, constant, and capable of extensive irradiation.

We have described the pattern of the fixed set in static persons. If, however, we evaluate the behavior of these people, their activity in performing tasks imposed on themselves, we must recognize that they have in this case to overcome an internal contradiction, fundamental in its implication. If the whole activity of static persons took place exactly along the line of their characteristic sets, it would undoubtedly present a completely different picture — we would see the true picture of behavior of the schizophrenic. In fact, this does not happen, and among the group of static persons, we often meet some with outstanding disabilities.

How can we explain this fact? What compensates for the peculiarities of static persons, making them useful members of society?

Objectivization is certainly responsible — a capacity which is noticeably strong in these people. They give the impression that their activity takes place mainly under the vigilant control of their consciousness. They must constantly inhibit the impulses of their own sets and choose the lines of their activity only after they have recognized the desirability of one particular course as a result of objectivization, after which, by efforts of will, they take steps to bring it to life.

Static persons are capable on the basis of objectivization of correcting that which is not quite normal in the structure of their being. Clearly, therefore, they experience their acts of objectivization much more acutely than persons with a dynamic structure. They themselves complain of the pain of these experiences, the great strain which they have to endure when they choose and operate a set which corresponds to what appears desirable to them on the basis of objectivization.

C. Variable Persons

Finally, let us turn to the investigation of the sets of a third group of subjects — the group of variable persons. It must be remembered, however, that this group includes at least two distinct subgroups. These are the variant of stable persons and the variant of labile persons. Let us now try to discover the most important distinguishing features of the sets of these groups.

Variable–Stable Persons. The first group of variable persons — the variable–stable group — differs from the rest mainly in one important characteristic. They attract attention by the highly developed strength of their needs, so that their behavior proceeds along the line of activation of sets for the satisfaction of these needs. During fixation of the set, the dominant role is played by the subjective factor — the strength of the needs seeking satisfaction. This relationship between the factors of the set — the predominance of the subjective factor over the objective — leaves its specific imprint on the whole typology of the set of the variable-stable person. Let us attempt to describe this set briefly.

In the first place we must stress its far-ranging variability. This means that the persons of this typological group rarely or hardly ever show signs of the constancy of their sets. Quite the reverse: Their sets vary from moment to moment, assuming the most varied form. Sometimes they are coarse and dynamic, at other times plastic and dynamic, sometimes they appear plastic and static, at other times coarse and static, frequently they are strictly localized, but sometimes they may be widely irradiated. In brief, the sets of persons of this group are extremely variable.

However, variability of the set also characterizes another

group of our subjects. The specific feature of this group, however, is the stability of its varying sets. This means that a variable set in these cases rigidly preserves its meaning — it remains variable within strictly defined limits. We therefore say that the variable set of this group of subjects is distinguished by its stability. If we express the degree of distribution of these signs among our subjects in figures, we must emphasize that in both cases its percentage reaches 100. Admittedly, each of these signs of the set is not always represented by the same numerical values in different sensory modalities (for example, stability of a set in the haptic sphere may be higher than in the optic), but the difference is not large enough to warrant special consideration.

Consequently, the distinguishing feature of the persons of this group is that they may react to a series of essentially different phenomena with identical sets, and, conversely, they may react to identical situations at different times with different sets. Let us assume, for example, that after 5 fixing exposures a subject has developed a coarse, static set. Sometime later it may be found that the same subject, in the same condition, exhibits a coarse, static or plastic, static set; it may also happen that no set whatever is fixed in this subject.

Without discussing other aspects of the set which differ by these same properties of variability and stability, I want to dwell on the power of objectivization shown by our variable-stable subjects. Experiments were carried out with 5 such subjects by the method of fixation of the set by reading and writing. A delay arising in the experiments caused the subject to objectivate the critical word, as a result of which he fixed it clearly enough as a Russian word. However, he was unable to write this word at once as a Russian word. He wrote it in a Latin transcription, as if it were a Latin word. In order to overcome the impulse of the fixed set and to put into operation the fact of objectivization, the subject had to make a very great effort.

Hence, we may conclude that the variable-stable subject readily carries out acts of objectivization. However, he cannot so easily develop his volitional acts which are essential before the results of his objectivization can be put into practice.

Variable-Labile Persons. The other group of variable subjects is composed of persons with variable-labile sets. The subjects of this group are characterized, first, by the weakness of their needs. In contrast to the first group of variables, fixation of their sets is determined by the priority of the situation, on the basis of which they develop and are confirmed. The external factor plays a more important role in the sets of these people than in other cases. This leaves a specific imprint on persons with variable–labile sets, distinguishing them as a special group differing from all other groups of our subjects.

What is the nature of the sets of variable–labile persons?

First, we are considering only a subgroup of variable persons. Consequently, there is no need to emphasize specially that the sets of these people are variable. The specific feature of their sets is lability, observed in almost 100% of all cases (actually 96%). The course of their fixed sets varies: Usually they are weak, but sometimes they may be strong and plastic and dynamic or coarse and dynamic, while in some cases they may be coarse and localized or coarse and irradiated. It may occasionally happen also that sets in this group of subjects are not fixed at all.

It is interesting that the excitability of the sets of these people is variable: It varies from subject to subject, and sometimes the results are very widely divergent. Under these circumstances, the set may be restricted to the region of its initial appearance; it does not spread to other sensory modalities, and it irradiates only slightly, although it is not always localized (indices of irradiation from 36% to 21%). Particular attention must be paid to the strong lability of our subjects; their fixed sets often remained in force not more than 1 hour, and sometimes even less.

The possibility of fixation of the set on the basis of imagination is not ruled out. However, such fixation is extremely weak and produces no more than one or two illusions. This is in harmony with their power of objectivization, which only comparatively rarely arrives at an active state in order to restrain impulsive acts of behavior.

The degree to which these distinctive features of the sets are reflected in the whole behavior of persons with variable sets can easily be seen. However, we shall not discuss this further, and we mentioned the problem merely as one requiring further detailed investigations.

2. Objectivization as a Force Independent of the Set

All these three groups of subjects differ from each other by the distinctive properties of their fixed sets. Whereas the largest of these groups — the group with dynamic sets — accounts for the great majority of our subjects, the other two groups — the group with static sets and the group with variable sets — consist of only a very few subjects.

Nevertheless, it must be recognized that people — ordinary toilers and creators of life — differ considerably from each other with regard to the types of their sets. However, this difference is not important. Whereas persons with dynamic sets must undoubtedly be regarded as most highly adapted, the other two groups play a no less important role. To judge by the type of sets, this would not be expected of them. In fact, however, the subjects of these groups, especially persons with a static set, usually cope well with their tasks and in some cases occupy high positions in society.

We have seen that this is explained by the activity of objectivization, which was present to some degree in all our subjects. This is particularly true of the last two groups. The power of objectivization, of course, is also present in dynamic subjects. However, in these subjects it is readily activated and operates without effort, so that it does not attract much attention. So far as the other two groups of persons are concerned, acts of objectivization, as we have seen above, take place with appreciable difficulty. This is because, by acts of thought and will developing on its basis, they have to overcome the strength of their natural impulses — the strength of the impulses of their static or variable sets — and to bring to life the desire for goal-directed activity, frequently in conflict with the impulses of these sets.

Hence, to judge by the results of this type of activity, no difference can be seen between persons exhibiting considerable variation in the type of their sets. All may achieve equally high degrees of productivity. This demonstrates the role of activity on the basis of objectivization, present in representatives of all these groups of subjects with different sets.

We may thus conclude that the power of objectivization liberates man from his direct dependence on natural sets and prepares him for independent, objective activity. It gives him the power of independent, objective action upon circumstances and the power to control them; it liberates man from direct, unconditional dependence on nature and assists him to become independent of its power and capable of controlling it.

However, man's natural features, in this case the features of his sets, continue to exist in him, but they continue to exist in a stereotyped form, so that they are no longer of decisive importance in human activity. At the level of objectivization, man becomes independent of nature and begins to control circumstances in accordance with features objectively associated with them.

However, the natural set in man continues to make itself felt. It is reflected in the subject's personal experience and it acts on him in a definite and appropriate direction. Persons with a static set, like those with a labile set, have their own personal experiences, which, in general, could be described as severe.

The questions arise: How constant and invariable is a subject's set? To what extent is it exposed to the influence of circumstances, and for this reason, are subjects with a particular set condemned to live with it for the rest of their life?

3. Constancy of the Set in Man

If we assume that man is born with a definite set, or acquires it once and for all during life, then there can be no doubt about the constant, unchanging nature of the set. If, on the other hand, the set is essentially dependent on the conditions in which it arises, if it is determined as fixed in these conditions, then we shall have to recognize that it can hardly fall into the category of unchangeable.

The mere enunciation of this question provides a clear answer. If sets are judged by the character of the essential conditions of their development, they cannot fall into the category of inborn entities, determined once and for all; for the concept of need, like that of environment, belongs to the group of phenomena dependent on the constantly changing conditions of existence of the organism.

Consequently, a simple analysis of the conditions of development of the set is sufficient to show that fatalistically predetermined sets, defined once and for all, do not exist.

Nevertheless, we must turn to observed facts in order to determined whether we may find data confirming the correctness of this view.

We must examine cases in which, because of the changing conditions of life, the subject himself has been transformed radically, in order to discover what has taken place with the typical features of the fixed set, whether they have remained untouched or have undergone specific changes corresponding to the actual typological changes taking place in the particular individual. We have made several observations showing that such cases actually exist

[61]. Some of the persons whom we studied have experienced during their lives events of major social significance, at the same time intimately connected with their own personal fate. These events were found to have played in the lives of these people the role of factors producing a profound reorganization in the structure of their personality: Subjects with a variable character became dynamic or static individuals, and, conversely, dynamic or static persons all at once became typical bearers of the characteristics of the variable man. It was not difficult to make these observations, for the subjects were investigated at first in prewar years, and again after the war, in which some of them had participated directly.

From this material we shall describe here one case which can be regarded as typical. One of these subjects — she was studied in detail in the years before the beginning of the Second World War — gave the impression of being a strong, confident person of a socially and individually altruistic temperament. She did her work energetically and resolutely, and usually completed it successfully. According to all the signs, she was a person with a decisive will and a solid character. She did not give way to her abstractions, however strong they were, and she was always ready to help those in need. To the outside observer she appeared to be a person with strong social and altruistic tendencies, ready to fight decisively and steadfastly to put them into practice. However, a closer look at our subject revealed that this was only the external appearance, for in fact she was really completely opposite to what she seemed. We saw in this case an almost complete divorce between human external appearance and internal nature.

Investigation of the fixed sets of this subject showed them to be coarse and static, irradiated, constant, and intermodally stable.

We happened to see the same subject 7 or 8 years later. During this period, a considerable change had taken place in her life; her husband had gone on active service and she was left alone. Caught up by these unexpected events, she soon became fully occupied in caring for her children, looking after their education and health, and thinking about her husband's return home. Her individualistic and egoistic tendencies grew weaker, and she developed into a strongly altruistic and socially responsible individual, having finally got rid of the second side of her character. The internal conflict had evidently disappeared without trace, so that we were left with a harmonious personality, quite unaware of her previous internal conflicts. To judge from these findings, the subject had passed through a critical stage, and her conflicting nature had now become one of complete harmony.

It is interesting to examine what had taken place with her sets. Had they remained the same, or had they also undergone a change?

Experiments showed that the sets of this subject had undergone considerable changes. No longer coarse and static, they had become plastic and dynamic. In this respect she had become quite a different person. So far as the other factors of her sets are concerned, these showed a smaller change. Her fixed sets were stable, irradiated, and intermodally constant, although within limits they showed traces of variability which, although insignificant, were nevertheless still detectable. Hence, we see from this example that the typological structure of human sets is not rigid and invariable. On the contrary, it may show substantial changes; for example, a subject's static sets may become dynamic. However, such changes demand crises in the subject's environmental conditions, changes far exceeding those of ordinary life.

There are many such examples. However, further investigations are necessary in order to shed more light on the conditions in which these changes may arise and on the directions in which they may go.

4. Scope of Sets in Man

Let us assume that an act of objectivization has been completed, and the process of thought arising on its basis has solved a problem in a definite manner. This is usually followed by stimulation of the set corresponding to the solved problem, and then by an effort for performing it, for putting it into operation. This is a purely human method of mental activity.

The question arises: Should this method be regarded as the only and essential method in the process of human mental activity, leaving no more scope for the direct activity of the set?

We concluded above, in our analysis of the problem of objectivization, that a subject resorts to this activity only when the need arises — when he is confronted with a problem that cannot be solved under the direct guidance of the set. But if this does not happen, if the problem can be solved directly on the basis of the set, then there is no need for objectivization and the subject need do no more than mobilize the corresponding sets.

Let us assume that a problem was solved for the first time on the basis of objectivization. In such cases, if the same or a similar problem appears later, there is no further need for objectivization and the problem is solved on the basis of the corresponding set. Once a set has been found, it may be revived directly, without the need for the objectivization which first produced it. This is how human sets appear and develop; besides the sets which can be summoned directly, there are others which must first be created by acts of objectivization.

The range of human sets is not restricted to those created by objectivization and by acts of thinking and will arising on its basis. We must also include those sets which were first built on the basis of objectivization of other subjects, for example, those endowed with creative gifts, and then transferred for general use as ready-made formulas, no longer requiring the direct participation of processes of objectivization. Experience and education, for example, are later sources of formulas of this type. A special period in human life is devoted to them — the school period, covering an increasingly longer portion of our life. However, the acquisition of complex sets of this type continues even after leaving school — human experience and knowledge is continually growing and developing.

Hence, the widening of the scope of human sets is in principle unlimited. Besides sets developing directly on the basis of actual needs and situations for their satisfaction, there are others either arising on the basis of objectivization by the individual himself or inculcated by education — the study of scientific and technological data.

These considerations show clearly how far apart are the ranges of the set in man and animals. Animals are unable to objectivate, so they cannot have sets created by this means. For the same reason, animals have no education, so that consequently they are unable to acquire sets developed by others. The animal is restricted entirely to the field of sets fixed in his own life, and these sets, moreover, are to a large extent diffuse, unlike those in man, whose sets differentiate further as they are differentiated more finely.

It cannot, therefore, be doubted that, although sets can be found in animals and serve as the basis for their activity, this does not mean that animals can be identified with man. The objectivization which arises in man, as a social individual, causes sharp changes in the composition and character of his sets. By lifting him to high levels of development, at the same time it raises the level of complexity, precision, and differentiation of his sets directly formed on the basis of actual situations.

Hence, fundamental differences are found between man and animals in the range of their sets.

VI. CONCLUSION

The foregoing facts may be summarized as follows: At the human level of development, we find a new and distinctive feature of mental activity which we describe as the ability to objectivate. This may be described as follows: When a person meets with a difficulty in the course of his activity, instead of continuing this activity in the same direction, he interrupts it for a short time in order to concentrate his attention on the analysis of this difficulty. He picks out from the chain of continuously changing conditions of his activity the circumstances of his difficulty; he holds each of these circumstances before his mental eye in order to perceive them afresh; and he thus objectivates them in order to reach the eventual solution of the problem of the character of his future activity.

The direct result of these acts interrupting our activity is that we can recognize them as such — we can identify them. When we objectivate something, we are able to realize that it will remain the same throughout the period of objectivization; it will remain itself. In brief, in such cases the principle of identity comes into force.

Once we develop the idea of the identity of an objectivated segment of reality with itself, there is nothing to prevent us from considering that we can re-experience this segment of reality any number of times, that throughout this period it will remain equal to itself. This provides the psychological basis, in the conditions of social life, ensuring that the segment of reality which has been objectivated and identified with itself can be designated by a definite name, or in other words, a basis for the creation and development of speech.

Furthermore, on the basis of objectivated reality and developing speech, the evolution of our thought takes place. This is a more powerful weapon for the solution of human problems — it decides what must be done in order to ensure the successful conclusion of temporarily interrupted activity. It gives instructions to the set which must be brought into operation by the subject for the successful conclusion of his activity.

In order to carry out the instructions of thought, however, a specifically human ability is required — the ability to carry out volitional acts — man must have a will, enabling him to resume his interrupted activity and to direct it into the channel corresponding to his goals.

Hence, we see that in the complex condition of human life, when difficulties and delays occur in human activity, the ability to objectivate is first brought into operation — a specifically human ability, on the basis of which subsequently arise identification, nomenclature (or speech), and the usual forms of thinking, followed finally, when the processes of thought are complete, by acts of will, setting the subject once more in the direction of his goal after the temporary interruption of his activity and ensuring the satisfactory attainment of his purpose.

Objectivization is a specifically human ability, and it forms the basis of the increased complexity and range of fixed sets in man. It must be remembered that a set arising on the basis of objectivization may in suitable conditions be reactivated directly, without any further participation of the act of objectivization. It forms part of the range of sets possessed by the subject and may be activated, like his other sets, without the need for objectivization. Hence, we can begin to understand how complex and rich the store of human sets may become, when they include those which at some time or other have been created on the basis of objectivization.

Set in Psychopathology

I. THE INTEGRAL BASIS OF PSYCHOPATHOLOGICAL PHENOMENA

1. Enunciation of the Problem

It is now firmly established that the basis of psychotic and psychoneurotic state is not a definite anomaly of some special character, not a disease of specific mental functions, but an integral process affecting the diseased personality as a whole. The search for pathological symptoms in the field of individual mental functions will not yield positive results. These functions remain basically unaffected; they function strictly in a definite manner: Sensory functions, just like other mental functions represented in man, remain precisely the same functions. It frequently happens that, in mental illness, the mental functions themselves remain unaffected and may function in basically the same way as in a normal state.

Evidently, it is not some individual function that is diseased, but something more fundamental, more integral, more personal in its nature. We may suppose that the disease affects not individual functions, but the personality itself which operates them. For this reason, it is not surprising that in the case of disease or simply of a depression of individual mental functions – sensory, motor, or even, perhaps, intellectual – the personality as a whole remains within normal limits.

Accordingly, the clearest forms of manifestation of a psychosis must be sought, not in individual mental or other functions of the sick person, but rather in the integral structure of his personality.

To find evidence for this hypothesis, we must study human sets in various psychotic states.

2. The Method of Study of Sets in Patients

The available methods of investigation of sets are mainly concerned only with their fixed forms. In this case, therefore, we shall necessarily be restricted to the study of the fixed sets of our patient. However, our methods, like any other experimental methods, assume that the subject is prepared to submit himself to investigation and to follow the experimenter's instructions. Normal subjects have no difficulty in this respect; they easily understand the problem and are prepared to carry out all demands of the experimenter. It is a different matter with mental patients. They cannot always understand the experimenter's wishes, and, therefore, experiments constructed in the usual manner, assuming that the subject is prepared to be investigated, are unsuitable. We must therefore ask how this difficulty can be overcome.

In experiments with animals, we make use of the fact that the presentation of food stimulates their activity to an adequate degree. Perhaps experiments with mental patients could be constructed in the same way. However, even in these conditions, success cannot always be expected in the case of an exacerbation of the patient's illness.

Until other opportunities are available, we therefore decided to limit ourselves to data which can be obtained from patients in a comparatively tranquil state. In this case, there is no need to make significant changes in the structure of our ordinary experiments; on the whole, they follow their normal course in these cases.

II. SCHIZOPHRENIA

In the first place, let us consider patients with schizophrenia. We have studied such patients previously [34]. It is only recently, however, that we have carried out systematic investigations of schizophrenia. At the present time, the whole staff of the Department of Psychopathology of our Institute is engaged with this problem, and we shall now describe some of the results of their work to try to solve the problem of the state of fixed sets in the schizophrenic patient and the role which they play in the disease.

1. Results of Experiments on Sets in Schizophrenics

The work of my colleague I. T. Bzhalava [16] has provided us with extensive material which is relevant to our problem. Altogether, 195 patients were investigated, of whom 32 (14.5%) were in a state which prevented them from taking part as subjects of the investigation. For one reason or another, familiar in the clinical study of schizophrenia (a state of acute psychotic disturbance, depression, etc.), it was impossible to get over to these patients the desire to follow the instructions of the experimenter, that is, to develop in them the "need" to see the problem in experimental conditions and to try to give a suitable reaction. Accordingly, these 32 patients had to be omitted from the total number of subjects.

Another group of patients would agree to obey the experimenter's instructions only at certain times, and usually the results which they gave could not be trusted. These patients (numbering 30, or 13.1%) were also omitted from the total number of subjects.

If we exclude the members of these two groups (62 patients) from the total of 195 subjects, we still have a large enough number of patients (133) to enable conclusions to be drawn from the results of investigation of the typical forms of sets in schizophrenics.

The first feature to be noted from the results of these experiments is the splitting of the fixed set of the schizophrenic, depending on the receptor organs used in each individual case. We know that in normal conditions the fixed set acts equally, regardless of which organ takes part in the reception of the stimuli acting upon the subject. In the unselected mass of subjects, it does not matter in which sensory sphere the fixed set is stimulated, haptic or optic. In both cases, practically the same number of illusions is obtained. Admittedly, in the optic sphere the number of cases of illusions is somewhat smaller than in the haptic, but normally this difference is so small that it can be disregarded.

In contrast, in experiments with one group of patients, this difference was so considerable that it could not be disregarded. For example, a group of 37 patients, (16.4%) showed such obvious dissociation of the set depending on the use of different receptor organs that due attention had to be paid to this fact. Whereas 100% of these subjects (all 37 patients) fixed their sets in the haptic field, only 16 patients (43.2%) did so in the optic field.

Hence, dissociation in the field of these two receptor organs is well established; the optic sphere, moreover, produced less reliable fixation of the set than the haptic sphere. We stress this

TABLE XVII

	Haptic set		Optic set	
	Absolute number	%	Absolute number	%
Excitability	28	75.6	5	37.5
Static or dynamic	32	86.5	4	25.0
Constancy	24	65.0	4	25.0
Localization	34	91.9	11	68.8
Rigidity	32	86.5	8	50.0
Coarseness	28	75.6	15	93.7
Stability	10	27.1	7	43.7

fact here especially in order that later, when we study sets in patients with epilepsy, we shall bear it in mind.

If we separate from the total number of subjects these 37 patients characterized by obvious dissociation of their sets in the optic and haptic spheres and examine all accessible aspects of the activity of their fixed sets separately, we obtain widely inconsistent data in certain cases (Table XVII); namely, the index of excitability of fixation of the sets in the haptic sphere is much higher (75.6%) than in the optic (37.5%). The difference between these two spheres is also evident from the point of view of dynamicity. Whereas the optically fixed set is dynamic in form in 75.6% of cases, the haptically fixed set shows a much smaller figure (13.5%). Conversely, it appeared in the form of a static fixed set much more frequently (86.5%).

Finally, these two sensory spheres differ sharply with regard to the constancy of fixation of the set. In the haptic sphere, this was found in 65% of subjects, compared to only 25% in the optic sphere.

Otherwise, as is clear from Table XVII, there is no significant difference between the indices of the fixed sets. If we characterize the fixed sets of this group of patients in terms of the forms predominant in these two sensory modalities, we would conclude that the sets are distinguished in these patients by their coarseness, rigidity, lability, and localization. So far as the remaining features of the set are concerned, — its excitability, static or dynamic nature, and constancy — in the haptic sphere it is characterized by high values and in the optic sphere by low levels of development.

Consequently, we would describe schizophrenics as a whole, as people with mainly a coarse, labile, localized, and fairly rigid set. If we add to this description the special features which are dominant only in the haptic sphere, then we would have to add to our definitition ease of excitability, constancy, and, in particular, the static nature of the fixed set.

We are left with the last and most numerous group of schizophrenic patients (96 patients, 42.6% of all cases), which differed significantly from that we have just examined, and which must therefore be treated specially. The first difference is that in this case, in contrast to the previous group, there is no dissociation between the states of the fixed set in the sensory fields which we investigated. The results relating to the set in the haptic sphere agreed in all important respects with the results obtained in the optic sphere. This is true, however, only if the degree of optimal fixation of the set was reached in both sensory modalities, and this usually required at least 15 fixing exposures. If the effect of fixation in the haptic sphere in these conditions reached 100%, in the optic sphere it did not fall below 81.2%. These figures are so close together that it may be concluded that in the conditions of optimal fixation, the sets in both these sensory fields give approximately equal indices.

The only difference found between these sensory fields concerned the degree of their excitability. The optic sphere was much less excitable than the haptic; with 2 exposures, a haptic set was fixed in 96.4% of all patients, but with the same number of fixing exposures, the total number of cases of fixation in the optic sphere did not exceed 58.3%. However, this is an unimportant feature and can disregarded. We will turn now to a detailed analysis of the properties of the set in the two sensory modalities and in other respects. The results of all the experiments undertaken for this purpose are given in Table XVIII.

The first feature which draws our attention is the extremely low level of the indices of the plastic and dynamic forms of set. The sets of the group of schizophrenic patients which we are studying were static (98% and 75%) and coarse (85.9% and 72%). At the same time, however, they were rigid (98% and 72%) and irradiated particularly intensively (100% and 100%). Less decisive results were obtained with respect to the constancy (76% and 55.2%) and stability (72.9% and 52%) of the sets in these schizophrenic patients.

Hence, we see that the fixed set of this particular group of

TABLE XVIII

	Haptic set		Optic set	
	Absolute number	%	Absolute number	%
Static	94	98.0	72	75.0
Dynamic	2	2.0	6	6.2
Coarse	82	85.9	69	72.0
Plastic	14	14.1	9	9.3
Constant	73	76.0	53	55.2
Variable	23	24.0	25	26.0
Stable	70	72.9	50	52.0
Labile	26	27.1	28	30.0
Irradiated	96	100.0	96	100.0
Localized	–	–	–	–
Rigid	94	98.0	69	72.0

schizophrenics must be described as coarse, rigid, static, and irradiated, and in most cases as constant and stable.

We thus find that our patients fall into two independent groups, differing considerably from one another. In order to obtain a clearer picture of this difference, let us compare the results obtained with these two groups, and let us confine our attention to the indices of sets in the haptic sphere (Table XIX).

The table shows that while the two groups of subjects show resemblances, there is also a considerable difference between them. This difference is concerned mainly with the indices of irradiation of the set. Whereas in members of the first group these indices are almost completely absent (8.1%), in the members of the second group irradiation is present without exception (100%). This is the most important difference observable between the members of these two groups of subjects.

At the same time, however, they differ in the stability of their sets. Whereas the subjects of the first group most frequently have labile sets (72.9%), the members of the second group show an almost equal degree of stability.

In all other respects, the sets of these two groups give approximately the same indices. Mention should be made of a comparatively great difference between the indices showing the presence of plastic and dynamic forms of sets. Whereas the subjects of the

TABLE XIX

	Group 1 (%)	Group 2 (%)
Dynamic set	13.5	2.0
Static	86.5	98.0
Plastic	24.4	14.1
Coarse	75.6	85.9
Constant	65.0	76.0
Variable	35.0	24.0
Irradiated	8.1	100.0
Local	91.9	–
Rigid	86.5	98.0
Stable	27.1	72.9
Labile	72.9	27.1

second group rarely showed the presence of such forms (14.1% and 2%), their incidence in the first group was much higher (24.4% and 13.5%).

What can be said about these two groups of schizophrenics? In the first place, the results with respect to irradiation of the set provide a sharp line of demarcation between them. Admittedly, in many other respects they differ very little from each other, but the difference with regard to irradiation is so considerable that it must receive proper attention. On the one hand, whereas all of the subjects of the second group show obvious irradiation of their sets, the first group of subjects, with the exception of 3 patients, were all characterized by localization of their sets. This phenomenon, of course, cannot in any way be regarded as normal, just as the presence of 100% irradiation of the set in the subjects of the second group is also abnormal. However, it is in sharp contrast to this same feature in the subjects of the second group, that is, the overwhelming majority of schizophrenic patients whom we have investigated.

If the essential importance of this feature of the sets in schizophrenic patients is recognized, then clearly the first group of subjects cannot be regarded as typical schizophrenics, and our attention must be concentrated on the second group. These can be regarded as the most typical schizophrenics, and the pattern of the dynamics of their fixed set can be regarded as specifically schizophrenic. Of the total number of patients studied in this case (133 persons), 96 (73%) belonged to this second group, that is, the group of true schizophrenics, and only 37 (27%) belonged to the first group.

Consequently, the great majority of the subjects investigated (73%) were characterized by rigid, coarse, static, stable, and irradiated sets. It may therefore be concluded that these are the forms of fixed sets which as a rule are found in schizophrenia.

Schizophrenia is thus based, among other things, on specific changes in the working of the patient's fixed set — a change toward the coarse, static, and irradiated nature.

This conclusion would be unquestionable did we not know of cases in which sets of this type are also present in persons who cannot be regarded on any pretext as true schizophrenics. We saw above, when we made a typological analysis of normal subjects, that a group of persons can be distinguished whose sets are coarse, static and iradiated, that is, show the same characteristics as the fixed sets of the great majority of our schizophrenics. However, this does not prevent them from behaving as healthy persons and conducting a perfectly normal life. This is the group which we call "static" subjects. Consequently, the forms of activity of the set of schizophrenics which we have discovered do not provide an adequate basis for their mental illness.

This means that we must search further for this basis, perhaps in a different direction. The truth is that the analysis of our patients' sets is not yet complete and we must now turn to the study of the specific, purely human form of set, to what we know as objectivization.

What do we know concerning the power of objectivization in schizophrenia?

2. Objectivization in the Schizophrenic

It cannot be considered that this power of objectivization has yet been studied adequately. Only the first steps have been taken to investigate it, but we must now use the results which have been obtained in order to attempt to answer this question.

The following method was used to investigate objectivization in the schizophrenic experimentally.*

The subject is given a series of separate words (8 in number) in a language which he knows. This is done in order to fix in him a

*V. Kvinikadze, The Act of Objectivization in Schizophrenics, 1947.

set based on reading in this particular language. The ninth word is given to him in the critical experiment. This is written in the same alphabet as the fixing words, but is taken from the vocabulary of a different language. Fixing words are then repeated (but 3 words in a row), followed by 2 critical words in each experiment. The words are presented by means of an ordinary mnemometer.

Clearly, the subject must be capable of following the experimenter's instructions and of carrying out the task accurately. The actual instructions are as follows: "Look here at this window! Words will be shown to you here. Read them carefully!" Eight fixing words are sufficient to fix a set based on reading in a suitable language, that is, the language of these fixing words. But the next word is taken from a different language than that on which the set has just been fixed. Consequently, there may be either an unhindered perception of the written image of this word, but without any realization of its meaning, or after it has been read there may be a short pause or interruption, so that the word is separated from the fluent series of fixing words and is made the object of special observation — it may be objectivated by the subject in order to discover what type of word it is.

Briefly, the experimental conditions are such that they may stimulate the act of objectivization in the subject, so that he is able to reflect on the nature of this word. However, as we have seen, the subject may behave differently: He may pass by the critical word without any special pause — he may avoid objectivating it. Clearly, the act of objectivization is essential for the accurate observance of these experimental conditions, and normal subjects, when tested in the same conditions, always make use of it. In the case of schizophrenic patients, these experiments are perfectly within their grasp, and consequently may be used to test their ability to turn, when necessary, to acts of objectivization and, on the basis of these, to acts of thought.

The subjects selected were patients with schizophrenia who were capable of carrying out all the instructions of the experimenter in accordance with the experimental conditions. We give below the results of tests of 52 patients, including some with catatonic and paranoidal schizophrenia, as well as hebephrenia, paraphrenia, and schizophrenia simplex.

Whereas only 9 patients (17% of the total number) possessed the power of complete objectivization, in all the other cases other variants of reaction to the experimental problem were encountered.

To understand these results, let us consider them in greater detail. All 9 patients who exhibited the power of objectivization gave the impression of normal individuals in these experiments. When they read the critical words — for example, a Russian word in a series of Georgian words — they stopped for a short time, repeated it twice or three times, and then eventually pronounced it in Russian. There was no doubt that they were able to objectivate it. The behavior of these subjects was essentially indistinguishable from the behavior of normal persons, the only exception being that the process of objectivization did not take place at once, but usually after a short yet distinct delay.

Among these subjects, 2 could be distinguished by the fact that they could not stop and concentrate on the material which they objectivated for any length of time. Their completed act of objectivization lapsed, preventing any possibility of the evolution of thought processes on its basis.

To this group could be added a further 7 subjects who could definitely perform the act of objectivization, but only in fits and starts; sometimes they were able to do so, sometimes they were not. There was no reason to deny them completely possession of this power; it was present, but they were not always able to activate it.

Turning now to another group of subjects, those who were completely unable to objectivate stimuli acting upon them, various groups can be distinguished, differing from each other in certain important respects:

(1). The first group of subjects (9 patients) could solve the experimental problem correctly and immediately; they clearly perceived the difference in language between the fixing and critical words, and recognized, for example, that one was Russian while the others were Georgian. In these experimental conditions, the sets of these subjects were not fixed, and for this reason they easily avoided making mistakes which were readily committed after fixation of the set.

(2). The second group of subjects (13 patients) were able to read the series of words presented to them without any delay, but it was clear that they did not recognize their meaning. If they happened to read one of the words incorrectly, or to distort it, they never noticed this and, without attempting to correct it, they continued their reading. Hence, these subjects read without the participation of consciousness, for reading is an active form of mental work requiring the understanding of meanings associated with the graphic representation of words.

(3). The next group of subjects (12 patients), as a result of the fixing experiments, achieved considerable fixation of their sets, which became definitely static in character. The critical words were perceived as words taken from the vocabulary of the same language as the fixing words. For example, the critical Russian word "gora" was perceived as the Georgian word "gora." These patients remained in the power of their existing sets and were unable to turn to acts of objectivization.

Strictly speaking, therefore, only 17% of our subjects were capable of objectivization in these experimental conditions. The rest were to one degree or another incapable of objectivization when required, and their thought processes could not develop on its basis.

The questions may arise here: Is this conclusion specific only for these experimental conditions? Is it because the reading of words is a complex act, especially when the words are taken from two different languages (fixing words from one language and critical words from another language, known to the subject)? It would therefore be desirable to repeat these experiments in conditions more within the subject's grasp.

Because of these objections, in the next series of experiments the patients were given a mosaic composed of 17 different parts, and they had to determine what it was. If the subject had difficulty in doing so, he was helped. When he gave a satisfactory reply ("Now I shall take it to pieces"), he was told, "You must put it together again!" After the pattern had been taken to pieces, unknown to the subjects, to the pile of pieces were added another 3 or 4 different pieces, very similar to the pieces belonging to the pattern. In these conditions, the subject had to try to put the pieces together again.

Do the conditions of these experiments satisfy the demands that the power of objectivization must be present? When the subject is asked to put the pieces together, he usually appears ready to do so. However, to solve the problem it is not sufficient to take any piece and place it in the proper place. Something more is required — he must take a special look at the piece, paying attention not only to its shape, but also to its size, in order to find the proper place for it. Thus, in order to solve the problem correctly, the subject must objectivate the individual pieces of the mosaic. Consequently, the experimental conditions require the power of objectivization. The subject must use it before he can solve the problem satisfactorily.

Since these experiments present no special demands on the subject's knowledge and skill, they differ from the reading experiments and may be regarded as more suitable when working with patients with mental diseases. They have the disadvantage, however, of stimulating the demand for objectivization too clearly; the experiments are so constructed that, from the very beginning, they compel the subject to examine carefully each individual piece before the proper place can be found for it in the mosaic as a whole.

What are the results of these experiments with our patients? As might be expected, the experiments strongly stimulated the patients to carry out objectivization. From the very beginning, they were forced to recognize the special features distinguishing each particular piece which determined its position in the mosaic as a whole. Most patients (42 altogether) belonged to this group of subjects. Considerably fewer failed completely to objectivate the pieces which they were given. They selected one particular shape and placed it wherever it happened to fall. We found not more than 3 such patients. Finally, 6 patients yielded no results from these experiments because of their negativism.

However, a careful analysis of the behavior of the first group of subjects shows that they did not all exhibit the same power of objectivization, and that most of them had a considerable defect in their activation of this power. It would be true to say that the power of objectivization remained adequately intact in only 15 of the subjects tested. Characteristically, however, subjects in this group with a distinct lack of confidence in their powers were comparatively numerous; they felt unable to solve the problem and thus differed from perfectly normal persons.

The next groups of subjects were still more abnormal. Several such groups can be distinguished by differences in the manner in which they attempted the solution of the experimental problems. Some nearly succeeded in solving the problems, but others were less successful. All, however, showed one special feature; they were unable to solve the problem despite the fact that the experimenter helped them. They complained that they were not used to the problem, or simply that they could not do it, that it was "intended more for an engineer than for them." "This is a job for an engineer," exclaimed some of our subjects. Perhaps there is some justification for this exclamation; perhaps in this case, in fact, some special constructive capacity is being tested, and not simply the power of objectivization. However, careful analysis shows that the experimenter in these cases was not concerned with establishing how correctly the patterns were assembled by the patients; they may not have been quite correct. He was concerned only with seeing how the subject performed acts of objectivization so that on their basis an attempt could be made to put the objectivated pieces together.

It must be remembered that these subjects sometimes include persons who can solve these problems without any apparent effort; they put the pieces together quickly and without hesitation. They can do this without the necessary acts of objectivization, and they impulsively carry out the task. These people are specially gifted, and might have become skilled craftsmen if they had applied themselves to the work. We are not concerned with them. We are merely discussing subjects who can solve problems only if they are capable of objectivating those aspects of the problem which are not given to them directly or indirectly. The problem thus consists, not of the assessment of the constructive powers of our subjects, but merely of the testing of their skill in performing certain aspects of the construction of an object which they have specially observed, so that their thought may evolve on this basis, and they may thus find the most suitable method of solution of the problem given to them.

We need not dwell specially here on all the attempts to solve the problems which our subjects made. We shall note simply that the commonest cases were those in which the patients, when attempting to solve the problem, were immediately held up by some insufficiently thought-out method of solution; it appears that the "determining tendency" appearing in these cases was too weak — it died away before producing a solution of the problem, giving way to direct, impulsive acts of behavior. The general impression was obtained that our subjects were unable to remain on the plane of objectivization long enough to be able to develop their powers of thought on its basis and to reach the satisfactory solution of the problem. They quickly slipped from this level. In such cases, it happened that they could not solve the problem; they grew tired, and eventually absolutely refused to make any further attempts in this direction.

Hence, we see that our patients in these experiments produced no new evidence to supplement that which we obtained in the experiment on reading.

What do these facts as a whole tell us? In both the first and the second cases, we were dealing with patients, admittedly few in number, who apparently succeeded in solving their problems correctly and comparatively easily. However, a careful examination of these cases revealed that the condition of these patients, although more or less adequate to the situation, was associated with the superficiality of their judgment, and that we were dealing with subjects who were not completely normal.

This is shown more clearly in the experiments with the remaining patients, who were quite unable to solve the problem given to them, although they appeared to be more or less prepared to do so. As we have seen, they received the experimenter's instructions, showed a wish to carry them out, but were unable to do so, mainly because they could not concentrate as they should on the problem. In brief, in all these cases, the power of objectivization was severely impaired.

Hence, we may conclude that in patients with schizophrenia there is a more or less obvious defect of the power of objectivization, and it must be assumed that this is one of the psychological causes of the distinctive deterioration of the patient's behavior.

Above, when we described the state of objectivization, we insisted that it is one of the most important aspects of human psychology. Analysis of the behavior of the schizophrenic shows that this power is undoubtedly defective in this case; the objectivization of the schizophrenic is definitely subnormal. However, if this is so, it means that profound changes must take place in the patient's mental life — his mind must work at a lower level than that of the normal person. We discussed above, the planes of mental life in general, and we saw that in man, because of the presence of this power of objectivization, several such planes must be distinguished. It thus becomes clear that the whole system of the mental life of man must become totally different — it must be completely reorganized if deprived of the power of objectivization. In cases of schizophrenia, this power is undoubtedly and severely affected, although this is not the only factor concerned.

Does this mean, however, that the schizophrenic, unable to objectivate phenomena and to develop his activities on a high level, is thereby reduced to the level of the normal mental life of animals? The answer to this question is obviously in the negative: The schizophrenic, of course, remains a man, but a man deprived of the specific feature of his mental life; he is now a sick, abnormal man.

It must be remembered that this disease is preceded by a lengthy period of normal development. Consequently, it affects what was a more or less normal person. On the basis of his established power of objectivization, his intellect developed — his power of logical thought — and then, or at the same time, his will — the basis of regulated, truly human behavior. When his power of objectivization began to be impaired, the normal working of all these systems based on objectivization naturally came to an end. Both intellect and will became forms of mental activity deprived of their usual normal basis. Bereft of this basis, both thought and will began to be manifested in pathological forms of activity, and this continued as far as the initial states of schizophrenia, in which they gradually disappeared and the patient became closer and closer to the state of the animal, although he can never be completely identified with it.

Further investigations are needed to show the extent, the direction, and the forms in which this basic change is reflected in the mind of the schizophrenic. They will also serve to concentrate attention on the solution of the problem of the specific nature of this change.

3. The Typological Basis of Schizophrenia

When we attempted to produce a typological classification of people leading a normal life, we concluded that they could be divided into three fundamental groups: dynamic, static, and variable persons. Strictly speaking, truly normal people should be regarded as dynamic, while static and variable people must be regarded as subjects with abnormal tendencies.

However, analysis of the behavior of these two latter groups shows that the course of their life is usually normal, and they thus remain perfectly adapted individuals. Moreover, the possibility is not ruled out that some persons may be found in these groups who, because of their talents, frequently stand above the average representative of the dynamic group. There is, therefore, no basis for excluding them from the category of normal subjects taking part in ordinary human life.

Yet this does not eliminate the question of the relationship between a particular type of normal person and a particular form of mental disease. This problem, in fact, confronts us in respect to schizophrenia. Do we find among healthy types, people who, by the structure of their character, stand particularly close to schizophrenia and who, should they become ill, must help to swell the ranks of the schizophrenics?

Earlier, when we studied human types, readily distinguishable from each other, we mentioned a group of subjects who could be described briefly as a group of persons with static sets. The study of their fixed sets showed that they are all characterized by rigid, constant, coarse, static, stable, and irradiated sets.

This means that the group of normal subjects with static sets are generally characterized by the same fixed sets as the main group of schizophrenic patients; their sets, as we have seen above, are also rigid, constant, coarse, static, stable, and irradiated.

Clearly, however, an essential difference between them can be identified. Analysis of subjects with static sets reveals that they are usually distinguished by a very marked degree of objectivization — the faculty on the basis of which the specifically human functions of intellect and will are based. The interference of these powerful forms of activity, resting on the basis of objectivization, gives the subject the possibility of exercising his normal control over his activities.

Let us assume, however, that this power of objectivization is impaired. In this case, we must also assume that the level of the intellect and will is also lowered. In these conditions, these functions are depressed and the subject possesses only those forms of fixed sets which in general characterize people in this group. Their behavior must therefore develop mainly on the direct basis of previously established fixed sets, that is, exactly as in patients with schizophrenia.

And so it becomes clear that the main force from which the ranks of the schizophrenics are filled is composed of persons with static sets.

III. EPILEPSY

From the results of our analysis of schizophrenia and the conclusions we have reached, we must now go on to consider whether a basis can be found for other mental diseases in the same direction as in the case of schizophrenia. In particular, we must do this in the case of epilepsy. At the end of his chapter on the nature of this disease, Gilyarovskii writes: "What is the relationship between the nature of the disease and the specific features of the character of the epileptic? There can be no doubt of the existence of a definite link between these aspects of the clinical picture. We may suppose that this character, like the specific features of their mental condition, provides the background on which a tendency toward convulsive forms of reaction develops.[27]

As a result of our elucidation of the problem of human typological structure, which we discussed above, we naturally are in full support of this proposed treatment of the question, and we may ask whether a basis for this disease in which we are now interested, may not be found in the same direction as that successful in the case of schizophrenia. In other words, are there specific changes in the sets of the epileptic which might be related to the nature of his disease?

1. The Fixed Set of the Epileptic

This question compels us to carry out our experiments on fixed sets with patients with epilepsy. This was done several years ago by our colleague I. T. Bzhalava [11], and we shall now discuss the main results of his experiment for they are directly relevant to this question.

Patients with genuine or essential epilepsy were investigated. The results of these experiments were not the same in all cases. It appeared that 3 groups could be distinguished among the patients, each of which showed its own special pattern of behavior of the fixed set. It was also found that these groups were very unequally represented numerically among the patients investigated; whereas one group comprised 72% of the total number of subjects, another accounted for 20%, and the third for only 8%.

What is the pattern of the fixed set in the first group of subjects? In other words, what is the pattern of the set in the vast majority of patients with epilepsy?

If we analyze the results obtained in accordance with individual aspects of sets, we obtain the following picture:

A. Excitability of the Fixed Set

This varied considerably from one patient to another. The first and principal group of patients, numbering 72 persons, (72%) gave a static set after 2 or 3 fixing exposures, but in 45% of all cases this set was plastic; that is, it changed its form, sometimes appearing as contrast illusions and sometimes as assimilative

*V. A. Gilyarovskii, Psikhiatriya 3:368 (1938).

illusions. This number of fixing experiments demonstrates to us the low threshold of excitability of the sets in this group of subjects. If we increased the number of fixing exposures to 5, in all cases a coarse, static set was obtained. A further increase in the number of fixing exposures to 15 hardly affected the picture — the set remained coarse and static. It was accordingly concluded that optimal excitability of the set in this main group of epileptics was secured by 5 fixing exposures.

The second group of patients — consisting of 20% of the total number of subjects — was distinguished by the fact that their lower threshold of excitability coincided almost completely with its optimal threshold; in this group of patients, sets were fixed as a result of 2 or 3 exposures, and this was quite sufficient to ensure optimal fixation. Hence, the level of optimal excitability was rather lower than in the first group of subjects.

Finally, the last 8 subjects showed a somewhat different picture: Three of them (37%) gave a typical fixed set after 2 or 3 fixing exposures. The remaining 5 subjects required at least 5 fixing exposures to produce the first signs of fixation, that is, its lower threshold, and the number of exposures had to be increased to 10 in order to reach the optimal threshold. This means that this group of patients occupies a special place — it includes subjects with different degrees of excitability of their fixed set; in some, it did not exceed 2 or 3 exposures, while in others it amounted to as many as 10.

Hence, we find that the great majority of our patients (72%) produced their typical form of fixed set as a result of 5 fixing exposures. The 2 remaining groups, which were very small, gave different indices, 2 or 3 and 10 exposures.

B. Extinction of the Fixed Set

The problem of extinction of sets as a result of reapplication of critical objects is of interest in its own account. In this case, as always, extinction of the set is measured by the number of critical exposures required to free the subject from his fixed set and to change to the adequate perception of stimuli acting upon him. Our experiments showed that the sets in all the epileptics were not equally extinguishable. Of our 3 groups of subjects, the first 2 groups gave absolutely identical indices; namely, if the subjects of these groups were given the optimal number of fixing experiments (usually 15 exposures), they all were found to produce a static set. This means that none of our patients was able to identify the equality of critical objects; that is, not one of them was able to free himself from the action of his fixed set and to perceive adequately the stimuli acting upon him. It must be remembered that this situation still applied whatever the number of critical exposures, at least up to 50 to 100 exposures.

The subjects of the third group were quite different. From the very beginning, they were capable of giving the right assessment of stimuli acting upon them. Instead of a static set, they were found to have a dynamic set, which gave them this possibility.

However, this group of subjects was very few in number, amounting to only 8 (8% of the total), whereas the other 92% all gave indices demonstrating the static character of their fixed set.

C. The Phases of the Fixed Sets of the Epileptic

As we know, the normal subject, during critical exposures, passes through a series of phases of change in his sets, until a new set, more adequate to the existing situation, takes over.

It is a different matter in cases of epilepsy. Experiments with these patients showed that in this respect they differ considerably from healthy persons. In particular, contrast illusions as a rule appear in epileptics from the very beginning. This means that their sets are fixed strongly despite the fact that the number of fixing experiments may not have been greater than 5. Despite the comparatively small number of fixing exposures, the phase of these illusions of contrast is unusually prolonged; it shows no significant change and continues to dominate the subjects in this form, without being replaced by some other set of different degree or quality.

Hence, fixed sets in epileptics are distinguished by their coarseness — they are always associated with contrast — and by their great strength, for they do not allow assimilative forms to appear.

This phenomenon holds good not only with respect to a particular group of subjects, but in relation to all three groups described above. Consequently, coarseness is the most general feature of sets in epileptics.

To sum up the results so far obtained, we may describe the epileptic as a person with a readily excitable, coarse, static, fixed set.

D. Irradiation of Sets

The degree of irradiation of sets is usually investigated as follows: Fixing exposures are carried out in one sensory modality (for example, the haptic), and the critical exposures in another (for example, the optic), and, depending on the results obtained, the degree of irradiation of the set from one sensory sphere to the other is judged. As a result of experiments of this type, the following conclusions were drawn regarding our epileptic patients: The first group of subjects showed hardly any cases of irradiation from the haptic sphere to the optic (not more than 4% of such cases in all). Rather more cases of irradiation in the opposite direction were found; the set irradiated from the optic region in 18% of subjects.

On the basis of these results, we may describe the sets in the first group of epileptics as mainly local, almost devoid of any property of irradiation.

The second group of subjects were the complete opposite to this; irradiation took place in them in all cases to the maximal degree (100%).

If these figures are compared with those obtained with the third group of subjects, it is clear that these groups approached each other nowhere as closely as this; irradiation from the haptic sphere to the optic was shown by 62.5% of subjects, and from the optic to the haptic by 50%.

Hence, in experiments on irradiation, for the first time we obtained results in which the second and third groups, which hitherto had always given completely contrasting results, came comparatively close to one another. The noteworthy feature of these two groups was the high ability of their sets to irradiate, whereas the first group, that is, the principal group of epileptics, differed radically from them by the well-defined localization of their fixed sets. We may say that this group of epileptics (72% of the total number of patients investigated) occupies a completely independent place, for irradiation of their sets to some degree or other was a common phenomenon in the two other categories of subjects.

The question naturally arises: How far is this ability widespread in epileptics? We are now able to measure the degree of localization of sets in still narrower limits; we can determine whether a set fixed in one of our paired organs (eye, hand, foot) will irradiate to its fellow organ.

These experiments are carried out as follows: The subject compares a pair of balls of equal weight but differing in size, but he does so in such a way that the solution of the problem falls on one hand. In the fixing experiment, he lifts at first the smaller ball with his left hand, and then the bigger one, in order to compare them (these experiments are repeated 15 times). Next, in the critical experiments, he receives equal balls one after the other in the right hand, with the object of comparing them successively. Approximately the same task is given in the optic sphere; the subject is given a pair of circles of different sizes one after the other tachyscoscopically, and he perceives them with one eye, since the other is kept closed at this time. The critical experiments then follow; in these experiments, the other eye takes part — the eye which was closed during the fixing experiment, and the subject after 15 such exposures compares a pair of successive equal circles. Similar experiments may be constructed for other sensory modalities.

The results of these experiments were similar to those obtained in the experiments described above.

In the first and most numerous groups of subjects, the set did not irradiate from one hand to the other or from one eye to the other. It remained confined to the limits of where it first appeared — the limits of the eye or hand participating directly in the fixing experiment.

Hence, we may conclude that the sets of the great majority of our subjects are not irradiated but remain strictly localized.

The subjects of the second group gave a completely different picture. In this case, as we saw above, a set fixed in one sensory region irradiated without hindrance into another region. For example, a set fixed in the haptic sphere spread easily to the optic, and vice versa. The same feature was observed with respect to the corresponding organs. In brief, the phenomonon of irradiation of sets was present in the second group of subjects (20% of the total number) without exception.

Finally, the third group of patients — the least numerous (8%) — showed a quite distinctive picture. First, in these experiments they did not always give identical results; that is, not one of this group of subjects gave the same indices in all variants of the experiments. If, for example, the experiment was one affecting corresponding organs (for example, the hands) and irradiation was found to take place, this does not mean that it would also take place if a different pair of corresponding organs or if different sensory spheres (for example, haptic and optic) were tested. Second, if, despite these differences between individual subjects, we nevertheless take into account all cases of irradiation of sets taking place in the experiments with this group of subjects, we find that their number amounted to 50% when both corresponding organs and independent organs were tested. These results show that the data obtained from this very small group of subjects may be disregarded when describing patients with epilepsy as a whole.

E. Stability of the Fixed Sets of the Epileptic

This characteristic feature – the well-marked immobility and rigidity – makes itself felt in all aspects of the action of the fixed set of the epiletic. This can be seen above in connection with its duration in time, and in connection with its stability. Suitable experiments can show how far it is characterized by this feature. Most interesting from our point of view is a more detailed knowledge of the main group of epileptics. The results of an experimental investigation of this group reveal to us the characteristic features equally applicable to all members of the group without exception. They show that fixed sets in these patients are dis tinguished by the high degree of their stability and by the almost complete absence of signs of variability; namely, if a fixed set in an epileptic is tested after 1, 2, or more days, it remains visibly unchanged. This may still be found weeks or even months after the day of fixation of a given set. Hence, fixed sets in epileptics are invariably a stable phenomenon, persisting for many months.

We are now speaking, of course, only of the largest group of these patients. Can the same remarks be expressed about the remaining two groups

So far as the second group of subjects is concerned, the results of experiments with these patients show no difference from the subjects of the first group; both gave sets of uniformly high stability in 100% of cases.

The situation is different with the third group, because they gave lower indices than all the rest of our subjects. Their sets proved stable in only 62.5% of the members of the group. The remaining 37.5% presented a more or less labile set.

Hence, we see that of our 100 subjects, 92 were characterized by strictly stable fixed sets, remaining active for many months.

F. Constancy of Fixed Sets in the Epileptic

The data concerning the stability of sets in epileptics clearly demonstrate their constancy. Nevertheless, a special investigation of this problem in our patients gave valuable results. We know that the constancy of a set is measured by the number of repeated experiments at definite intervals of time (usually every 24 hours) in which the set remains unchanged in every respect. In this case, experiments in which 15 fixing exposures were given were repeated 7 times every 24 to 48 hours. The results are given in Table XX.

Clearly, the subjects of the first group, that is, our principal group, retained their fixed set without exception for 5 days. The same result was obtained with the second group of subjects; in this respect, they were identical to the first group. The third group gave different results. The odd feature here was that whereas 100% of subjects used the same set after 24 hours as before, after 2 days this no longer applied. The number of such subjects fell suddenly to 62.5% (6 patients), at which level it remained until the end of the experiments, if we disregard the third day, when the percentage of subjects again rose to 75%.

G. Rigidity of Fixed Sets in Epileptics

How rigid were the fixed sets in our patients? A rough answer to this question is given by the results we have already obtained during the investigation of other features of sets in epileptics. However, it has also been analyzed in special experiments, and in order to have more accurate data we will now turn to the results of these experiments [11].

In all these groups of our subjects the number of critical exposures was increased to 100. The first and principal group gave an uninterrupted series of usual reactions (contrast illusions), and not one of these patients gave a reaction of equality or an assimilative illusion. This means that the rigidity of the fixed set in epilepsy is well established, yielding exceptionally high indices.

The same results were obtained in experiments with the second group of patients. However, the third group gave a different picture; despite a large increase in the number of critical exposures in 5 of 8 patients, the nature of the reactions remained unchanged

TABLE XX

Types of set	1 day	2 days	3 days	4 days	5 days
I	100	100	100	100	100
II	100	100	100	100	100
III	100	62.5	75.0	62.5	62.5

and the sets continued to be coarse and dynamic throughout. However, in 3 subjects, the picture was slightly different, with an increase in the number of fixing exposures to 30; to begin with, for a short time they gave a continuous series of illusions of contrast, but eventually (after 30 to 50 such experiments) they returned to their usual type of reactions.

Hence, in this case also this group of subjects continued to occupy an exceptional position, whereas all the rest presented an exceptionally rigid fixed set.

2. Specific Features of the Fixed Set in the Epileptic

To summarize the foregoing remarks and to try to describe the state of fixed sets in the epileptic, we must first study the question of the significance of the results obtained with three groups of subjects for our purpose.

Since the results given by the third group in nearly every respect differed from those obtained with the other two groups, and since this group included only a very small number of patients (not more than 8), this material can be disregarded when defining the state of the set in the epileptic.

So far as the second group of subjects is concerned, although admittedly in many ways they gave the same results as the first group, in one very important respect they differed radically from it. The fixed sets of this group of subjects were irradiated, whereas those in the first group of subjects did not have this property and were purely local in character. This extreme difference between the two groups in this fundamental respect compels us, when describing sets in epileptics, to disregard also the results obtained with the second group of subjects (20%).

We are left with the first group of patients (72% of the total number of subjects), presenting a surprisingly uniform and harmonious picture of their fixed sets. There is reason to suppose that this is the typical picture of the set of the epileptic. In general, it can be described as a comparatively easily excited, coarse static, local, constant, stable, and rigid fixed set. Since the most characteristic features of the set of the epileptic are its coarseness, its static quality and its localization, we may conventionally describe this set by these three terms; we may say that the epileptic has coarse, static, local fixed sets.

3. Typological Basis of Epilepsy

The question arises: Can we find normal people who are characterized by the same coarse, static, local sets as epileptics?

If we turn to the corresponding results, we shall find material concerning the static fixed set of the group of static persons [61, p. 345 ff], showing a very close resemblance to the picture of the fixed set of the epileptic. This is one of the groups of persons characterized by a conflicting personality and a static set, that is, the group of epileptoids. The fixed set appeared identical with those of the epileptic—coarse, static, localized, comparatively easily excited, constant, and stable. Strictly speaking, there is no visible difference between the sets of persons of this group and the group of epileptics.

Nevertheless, they are still far from being epileptics. In the first place, they never have epileptic seizures with their characteristic motor manifestation. Second, they are normal members of society, useful workers, sometimes reaching positions of high social importance. Many members of this category of people may be named among the ranks of outstanding artists and historical figures.

Consequently, it must be recognized that the basis of epilepsy must not be sought in the direction of the existence of seizures. Seizures of this type may also be found, for example, in cases of hysteria — a disease very different from epilepsy. We must conclude that in discussing seizures we are discussing a pathological phenomenon which cannot be regarded as specifically epileptic.

Without touching on the true nature of this disease, we may draw attention to some of the psychological peculiarities found in epileptoids and epileptics. In the first place, our interest lies in the higher, purely human mental functions — the intellect and the will.

There is no need to make a special experiment analysis of these mental forces in epileptoids. Among them can be named people with a high level of intellectual and volitional powers; there are many outstanding historical figures belonging to the class of epileptoids. Consequently, we must accept that the level of development of their objectivization, on the basis of which their outstanding intellectual and volitional powers may act, is high.

The situation is different with the true epileptic. Analysis of his intellectual and volitional data, in contrast, shows that in this respect the epileptic is at a much lower level of development. Facts confirming this conclusion are to be found in I. Bzhalava's dissertation [11, p. 401 ff, pp. 529-578]. An experimental analysis of the conceptual thinking of epileptics showed that this fundamentally important function is considerably depressed in these patients. However, the analysis of volitional acts, as might have been expected, does not provide us with better results. Without discussing the concrete picture of the will of the epileptic, at this point we shall merely state the fact that it is weakly developed. The epileptic is known as a person endowed with sthenic, aggressive emotions of unusual obstinacy and firmness, a person who will not hesitate to take steps possibly endangering his own life. This simply confirms the low level of development of his volitional qualities. Everything goes to show that he is governed by direct impulses, and not by rational will, the essence of which amounts, among other things, to the ability to control and direct these impulses, but not to submit to their direction.

Briefly, the intellect and will of the epileptic carry the imprint of obvious depression. On the other hand, there may be moments in the life of the epileptic when he is capable of high flights of thought and of volitional activity. We may imagine that in the epileptic, as in patients with other diseases, it is not so much the direct strength of thought or will that is primarily affected as the power of objectivization, the basis for both these activities.

In this case, the main cause of the absence or depression of the activity of the intellect and will of the epileptic must be sought in a disturbance of the power of objectivization. For some reason or other, which we shall not discuss here, the act of objectivization is impaired and, as a result of this, inertia of the intellectual and volitional powers of the individual develops. Consequently, his behavior, without the guidance of these higher forces, remains in the power of the sets specific to the particular personality. From then on, his behavior develops unhampered under the guidance of these sets. In the case of epilepsy, the basis of behavior becomes the coarse, static, localized, fixed set, and the patient is unable to correct his behavior under the guidance of his intellect. In schizophrenia, on the other hand, as we have seen above, as a result of the loss of the normal activity of objectivization and of the intellect and will based upon it, the activity of the fixed set is brought directly into play, characterized in this case by its coarseness, its static nature, and its irradiation.

IV. BORDERLINE STATES

Of the so-called borderline states, we shall confine our attention to the analysis of psychasthenia (of the type of inborn pathological states) and hysteria (of the type of reactive changes associated with mental experiences). As we know, these states, even "when associated with phenomena of very great intensity, are not diseases in the true sense of the term" (Gilyarovskii). On the other hand, they can be regarded still less as phenomena of normal, healthy states. Let us now analyze the sets in these states [37].

A. PSYCHASTHENIA

1. Fixed Sets in Psychasthenia

To determine the nature of the fixed sets in psychasthenia, an experimental analysis has been made of this state [37]. The results may be summarized as follows:

A. Excitability of the Fixed Set

Among psychasthenics, only a very small number of patients is found (not more than 12%) in whom sets can be fixed by 2 or 3 exposures of our ordinary experimental balls. The great majority of patients (88%) in this state cannot be influenced by this number of exposures. It may accordingly be concluded that the sets of psychasthenics are comparatively difficult to fix; 2 exposures, in any case, are rarely adequate for this purpose. Consequently, we may say that the excitability of the fixed set of the psychasthenic is very low, and, in order to reach its optimum, the number of fixing exposures must be increased considerably.

B. Rigidity of the Fixed Set in the Psychasthenic

This is characterized by very low indices. The first phase (that is, the phase of illusions of contrast) rarely occurs, and, if it does, it is extremely short and is soon replaced by the next phase in which assimilative illusions are predominant.

C. Coarseness of the Set

This observation clearly shows that the set of the psychasthenic possesses low plasticity; it does not pass through a series of stages of gradual extinction, but remains from the beginning at one particular phase. Hence, the fixed set of the psychasthenic must be defined as coarse and rigid in form.

D. Dynamicity of the Set

The next feature of the set in the psychasthenic is its dynamic quality. It is difficult to fix, but once fixed it retains its initial form, but it is then quickly discarded and replaced by an adequate, unfixed set.

E. Irradiation of the Set

The irradiation of this type of coarse fixed set, difficult to excite and of low rigidity, can hardly be particularly high. Experiments show that, in fact, the fixed set of the psychasthenic irradiates only to an insignificant degree; irradiation of sets was found in only 8% of our subjects. In the rest, it could not be detected experimentally. It can be concluded that in our experimental conditions the fixed set of the psychasthenic is definitely local in character.

F. Constancy

The fixed set of the psychasthenic was found to be very constant; once excited, it preserved the same form of a coarse, dynamic, local, fixed set, difficult to excite and of low rigidity. This property of the set in the psychasthenic deserves special attention, for it reveals the specific feature distinguishing the psychasthenic from patients with the other type of borderline state — the hysteric. We shall turn to this point again below.

G. Lability of the Set

Finally, the set of the psychasthenic is highly labile; in 80% of patients tested, the sets were found to be unstable. They quickly died away and were replaced by adequate sets.

Hence, it may be concluded that the fixed set of the psychasthenic is difficult to excite, weak, coarse, dynamic, local, constant and labile.

If we examine this picture of the fixed set of the psychasthenic carefully, we may ask: Can all these properties be regarded as specific features of the fixed set of the psychasthenic or must they to some extent be attributed to difficulty in the process of its fixation?

We pointed out above that this process is usually preceded by a more or less prolonged period of differentiation of the set; existing initially in a more or less diffuse state, the set must first become differentiated, must be defined as an individual and concrete state of the subject, and only then may it become fixed in this form. What happens in the case of the set of the psychasthenic? Is it differentiated adequately from the beginning, so that in the fixing experiment we are in fact concerned with its fixation or is the problem rather one of its differentiation?

Observations show that for the set of the psychasthenic to become fixed, a comparatively large number of fixing exposures is necessary. Remembering that the first phase — the phase of contrast illusions — is usually not present in these patients, it is clear that, as mentioned above, their sets undergo only weak fixation. The same conclusion can be drawn from other findings which have been mentioned above. Evidently, there is absolutely no doubt that the set of the psychasthenic is qualified by a weak degree of fixation.

It must be accepted in this case that, during repetition of the fixing exposures, many of these are utilized in the differentiation of the initially diffuse set, and that in any event a strong degree of fixation cannot be achieved. However, if this is so, we can define the psychasthenic as a person with a weakly differentiated set which remains, for this reason, difficult to excite, weak, local, and labile.

2. Objectivization in Psychasthenia

Before we can understand the psychasthenic, we must examine his objectivization. Observation of the psychasthenic shows that he is usually under the power of one of his ideas — the one which troubles him first and foremost. Dominance by obsessive ideas may perhaps be one of the most characteristic features of the psychasthenic. He is constantly in doubt about the correctness of his actions and in an irrepressible state of vigilant self-examination. The impression is created that the psychasthenic has no precise, clearly defined sets on the basis of which he can develop his arbitrary activity. The low level of differentiation of his sets is the main handicap preventing him from developing his volitional activity. This basic characteristic of the psychasthenic — the weak development of his volitional acts — rests on the inadequate differentiation of his sets. Despite the high degree of development of his objectivization, the psychasthenic has little success in constructing the pattern of his activity on the basis of its results, because these results are diffuse and unsuitable as a basis for volitional activity. The psychasthenic lacks confidence in the correctness of his acts, confidence which usually grows on the basis of definite sets, and which is absolutely essential for the transformation of these acts into life.

The intellect of the psychasthenic does not suffer the same fate. On the contrary, the presence of his power of objectivization provides an excellent basis for its activity, which frequently, perhaps even more often than is in fact necessary, stops to solve the problem of how to behave in a particular case. Although a satisfactory solution to this problem is often achieved, because of lack of confidence, growing on the basis of definite and appropriate sets, the psychasthenic is unable to dwell on anything in particular, and he feels compelled to seek other methods of solving his problem, or, at the actual moment of decision, he puts it off to a future occasion.

Consequently, the psychasthenic's lack of will also affects the productivity of the often high degree of development of his intellectual powers. It cannot give them the necessary rigidity for their transformation into life. It must be assumed that the basis of this defect lies in the weakness of confidence, resulting from the inadequate differentiation of the set in the psychasthenic.

Hence, the fundamental phenomenon determining the weakness of the mental activity of these patients is the inadequate differentiation or the high level of diffuseness of their sets, giving rise to lack of confidence, weakness of volitional acts, and instability of intellectual decisions.

B. HYSTERIA

1. The Fixed Set in Hysteria

Let us now turn to the problem of hysteria — a problem which has been studied from the earliest times and from the most widely separated points of view. We must discuss it from the standpoint of our concept of the set. We must determine the state of the set in hysterical patients, the way it works, and the distinctive features which it shows.

It may be concluded from a special investigation of this problem [33] that hysteria differs substantially from other diseases, in particular, in the great variability of the fixed set. In the hysterical subject, it is difficult to find a form of activity of the fixed set which can be expected from him in every case. On the contrary, a much more characteristic feature is the gradual fluctuation between the possible forms of set.

Nevertheless, there is a definite amplitude which characterizes these fluctuations, and our first task must be to establish its limits.

The fixed set of hysterical patients in the period of treatment is characterized by one essential feature; that is the fact of its constant variation within wide limits. To illustrate this point more clearly, we give below an account of one of our patients.

Patient D. L., female, aged 23 years, average education. She had attacks daily. Tests of her fixed set (December 19, 1935) showed it to be coarse, static (30 haptic illusions of contrast), and strongly irradiated (15 similar illusions of contrast in the optic sphere).

On December 23, 1935, she felt better. Tests showed the presence of a coarse, static set in the haptic sphere, which did not irradiate to the optic; she now reported the optic equality of the critical objects.

On December 25, 1935, she felt better. Although her attacks continued, they were not so frequent as before. Experiments with sets revealed plastic illusions, culminating in the fact that she reported the equality of the critical objects.

On December 27, 1935, she felt better. The experiments gave the same results as 2 days before.

On December 29, 1935, she had had no attacks for 2 days. She felt fit. The experiments gave approximately the same picture as on the last two occasions.

On January 1, 1936, she had not felt well the day before, but had no attacks. The experiments showed that her set was not fixed this time, and critical objects were perceived as equal.

The day previous to January 7, 1936, she had had a long attack, lasting about 2.5 hours. During the attack, she heard someone speaking to her in a loud voice, but it was difficult to understand. Her set was coarse and static, with brief irradiation into the optic sphere.

Tests continued on this patient until January 29, 1936. On January 14, 16, 20, and 25, she stated that she had had no attacks and that she felt better.

The experiments show that on some days she had a definitely plastic, dynamic set, which irradiated from the haptic to the optic region. On other days, when the attacks were repeated almost daily, she showed a variable picture of her fixed set.

On the whole, throughout the period of observation, this patient showed the following picture of constant variation of her fixed set:

A. After a series of attacks the previous day, she showed symptoms of a depressive state with headaches. While in this state, she gave a long series of illusions of contrast, with continuous irradiation from the haptic to the optic sphere; that is, her set was coarse, static, and irradiated. In this state, she resembled persons with a static set and phenomena of conflict. However, this was only after repeated attacks, while on the road toward an improvement in her state. It often happened that the set in this patient was not fixed at all.

B. In the same state, but in a milder form, and when the patient began to feel better, her set changed. It still had the same coarse and static form, but did not irradiate from the haptic to the optic sphere; it gave way almost immediately to adequate perception — the impression was gained that in this case something like the fixed set of the epileptic was seen.

C. Finally, after a series of days of freedom from attacks, the patient felt cheerful; her mood became comparatively lighthearted, and in this state she gave the fixed set of a normal, well-adjusted person. She had a set of plastic, dynamic type, irradiating readily from the haptic to the optic sphere.

These are the results obtained with one of the patients, and they do not differ essentially from those obtained with other hysterical subjects in this series.

We can thus repeat that the characteristic feature of hysterical subjects is the variability of their fixed set, taking place within wide limits. Depending on the patient's condition, it may be the perfectly normal set of a dynamic person, or the pathological set of the epileptic with a local and, in some cases, an irradiated fixed set.

We have described the set of hysterical subjects. We have seen that hysteria differs from the other pathological states we have described by the great variability of the fixed set and by the absence of its constancy, demonstrated by all the pathological cases analyzed above.

The variability of the fixed set, in close correlation with the variability of the behavior of the hysterical subjects, is one of the most characteristic features of hysteria.

However, hysterical subjects also show several other distinctive features which must also be studied to complete our picture of this disease. We must first discover whether the hysteric can stimulate his set on the basis of imagination.

2. Stimulation of Set on the Basis of Imagination

Special experiments on this subject provide a conclusive answer [24]. They show that, with respect to the subject under discussion, hysteria is characterized by specific indices which differ significantly from those given by normal, healthy subjects, and also from those found in patients with other pathological states.

If we compare the results of experiments to stimulate the fixed set on the basis of ideas in normal persons with those obtained with our hysterical patients, we find that the latter are far superior to the former in many respects. For instance, hysterical subjects develop a set on the basis of an imagined idea much more easily than normal subjects, and, what is particularly interesting, this set is appreciably stronger than in healthy persons.

The extent of the difference in this respect between the patients and healthy subjects is clear from the following facts: Whereas 60% of our hysterical patients developed a strong illusion of the set in response to an imagined idea in the haptic sphere and 46% did so in the optic sphere, illusions of this type were detected in only one healthy subject (17%).

Sets stimulated on the basis of imagination proved almost as strong in the hysterical subject as sets stimulated by the action of a concrete situation. If we consider other facts concerning the fixed set, we find the same results in nearly every line of its development. Accordingly, we may conclude that a set stimulated in an hysterical subject on the basis of his ideas is not noticeably weaker than a set produced on the basis of a concrete situation. This confirms the important role of imagined ideas in the mental activity of hysterical subjects.

The question naturally arises: What is the nature of this idea? We mentioned above that two fundamentally psychological aspects of this problem must be distinguished. First, there are "ideas" which exist in the undifferentiated or almost undifferentiated plane of our consciousness. These ideas are not differentiated from other aspects of its activity and, in particular, from what we term "perception." We find such "ideas" in dream states. However, we find the second type of "idea" in our specific experiences, which can be easily differentiated from "perception" and which is independent of the action of concrete stimuli. We have proved above that this differentiation of "ideas" takes place only on the basis of objectivization, that is, of a process confined to man.

Bearing in mind these two definitions of the concept of idea, and if we examine the "ideas" of the hysterical subject on this basis, we must realize that these are his experiences existing in the first, relatively undifferentiated plane of consciousness. Clearly, therefore, the set of hysterical subjects, arising on the basis of these "ideas." can hardly be distinguished from sets acting on the basis of concrete perception, because these "ideas" are not mental states differentiated psychologically from perception.

Hence, we may conclude that the ideas of hysterical subjects are experiences undifferentiated from concrete perception — experiences other than those which, as we mentioned above, exist in the ideas of our dreams. We must therefore recognize that the existence of "ideas" in hysterical patients by no means implies acceptance of their power of objectivization. The "ideas" of hysterical subjects are elements of consciousness which are in no wise objectivated. In periods of relapse, the consciousness of the hysterical subjects sinks into a state which closely resembles the state of our consciousness during dreams.

The question naturally arises: What is the relationship between a set stimulated by an imagined idea and the actual fixed set of the hysterical subject? We have seen that this latter is distinguished by the extreme variability of the forms of its manifestation. Is this feature reflected in the phenomena of the set fixed on the basis of the imagined idea? If we examine the facts relating to this type of set, we find that all the special features of the set fixed in actual conditions are repeated almost without exception. Hence, we must recognize that the feature of variability continues to be a characteristic property of the set of hysterical subjects.

To sum up, we may describe hysterical patients as persons with extreme variability of their sets, which may readily be fixed both on the basis of perceptions and on the basis of ideas only slightly differentiated from them.

3. The Premorbid State of the Hysteric

Let us now consider the premorbid state on the basis of which hysteria usually develops. Earlier in the book, during the investigation of the fundamental typological units, we had the occasion to analyze the type of what we describe as variabile–labile persons. We saw then that the variability and lability of the fixed set, and equally the frequent occurrence of cases in which the set could not be fixed, are the most characteristic features of persons of this type. Just as in hysterical subjects, the fixed set of these persons is lacking in constancy; it varies from case to case, and shows a definite tendency toward rapid extinction, and sometimes toward the total impossibility of fixation. Hence, if we compare the distinctive features of the set of variable–labile persons with the properties of the set in hysterics, the close resemblance between them is quite clear. Furthermore, the impression is created that in fact there may be no significant difference between them.

However, if we consider acute cases, the hysterical subject differs essentially from a person of variable–labile type. Whereas the latter is an ordinary, healthy person, leading a normal and, in some cases, productive life, the hysterical subject is definitely a sick person, who, when his condition relapses, leaves the ranks of the normal individual and becomes the subject of special observation and care of those around him.

What is responsible for these fundamental changes in the state of the variable–labile person? Without mentioning other, and possibly very important factors, I shall dwell only on one. Variable–labile subjects, like all variants of the conflicting type of persons, remain at the level of normal living beings insofar as they are capable, if need be, of regulating their behavior from the standpoint of objectivization, which to some extent they all succeed in doing; at decisive moments of their life, they mobilize their strength for this objectivization, and, on its basis, they develop suitably adapted forms of activity. During attacks of hysteria, however, this possibility is absent, and the behavior of the subjects is based on natural, impulsive sets. In this case, we see the picture of hysteria, in the precise meaning of the term.

Bibliography Concerned with Problems of Sets

1. E. K. Abashidze, Extinction and Stability of the Experimentally Fixed Set (1944).
2. E. K. Abashidze, The Factor of Satiety in the Action of Experimentally Fixed Set (1947).
3. E. K. Abashidze, A Method of Measurement of Excitability of the Experimentally Fixed Set (1946).
4. A. M. Avalishvili, "The Intermodal Constancy of Types of The Fixed Set," Tr. Gos. Univ. 17 (1941).
5. A. M. Avalishvili, "The Fixing Role of Critical Exposures," Psikhologiya 1 (1942).
6. N. G. Adamashvili, The Fixing Action of Illusory Perception (1937).
7. N. G. Adamashvili, "Intermodal Transposition of Illusions of the Set," Tr. Tbilissk. Gos. Univ. 17 (1941).
8. N. G. Adamashvili, "Irradiation and Rigidity of the Set," T. Tbilissk. Gos. Univ. 17 (1941).
9. N. G. Adamashvili, "The Fixed Set of Lower Monkeys," Psikhologiya 5 (1948).
10. I. T. Bzhalava, "Distinctive Features of the Fixed Set in Genuine Epileptics," [candidate dissertation, 1940].
11. I. T. Bzhalava, "The Psychopathology of Epilepsy (Clinico-Psychological Investigation)," [doctoral dissertation, 1944].
12. I. T. Bzhalava, "The Fixed Set in Cases of Simulation," Absts. Proc. Conf. Division of Social Sciences, Acad. Sci. Georgian SSR (1942).
13. I. T. Bzhalava, "Traumatic Neurosis," Tr. Inst. Functional Nervous Diseases, Vol. 2 (1945).
14. I. T. Bzhalava, "The Psychopathology of the Will," Absts. Proc. Conf. Division of Social Sciences, Acad. Sci. Georgian SSR (1944).
15. I. T. Bzhalava, "Diagnostic Value of the Fixed Set in Hysteria and Epilepsy," Psikhologiya 3 (1945).
16. I. T. Bzhalava, The Fixed Set of Schizophrenics (1947).
17. I. T. Bzhalava, The Fixed Set of Maniacal Patients (1940).
18. I. T. Bzhalava, "Pathology of the Fixed Set in Neuroses and Psychoses," Absts. Proc. Conf. Evacuation Hospitals in Transcaucasia (1944).
19. I. T. Bzhalava, "Typology of Post-Concussive Reactions," Psikhologiya 2 (1943).
20. I. T. Bzhalava and A. R. Luriya, The Fixed Set in Local Lesions of the Cerebral Cortex (1949).
21. I. T. Bzhalava, "The Fixed Set and the Speech Areas of the Cerebral Cortex," Psikhologiya 4 (1948).
22. I. T. Bzhalava, "The Psychopathology of the Frontal Cortex," Tr. Med. Inst. Tbilisi (1948).
23. A. T. Bochorishvili, "Analogue of the Illusion of Weight in a Region of Pressure," Izv. Tbil. Gos. Univ., 7 (1927).
24. E. A. Vachnadze, Distinctive Features of the Set on the Basis of Activation of the Imagination in Hysteria (1946).
25. E. A. Vachnadze, The Fixed Set of Schizophrenics on the Basis of Activation of Imagination (1947).
26. V. L. Kvinakadze, Objectivization in Schizophrenia (1944).
27. E. D. Kezheradze, "Rational Material and Repetition," Psikhologiya 1 (1942).

28. E. D. Kezheradze, "Development of Attention in Preschool Age," Psikhologiya 4 (1947).
29. E. D. Kezheradze, The Role of Objectivization in Memorizing (1946).
30. E. D. Kezheradze, The Development of Memory in Preschool Age (1947).
31. A. R. Luriya and I. T. Bzhalava, The Fixed Set in Lesions of the Cerebral Cortex (1948).
32. K. D. Mdivani, Peculiarities of Behavior of Schizoid Children (1931).
33. K. D. Mdivani, "The Fixed Set in Hysteria," Tr. Inst. Funk. Nervnykh Zabolevanii 1 (1935).
34. K. D. Mdivani, The Fixed Set in Schizophrenia (1936).
35. K. D. Mdivani, The Fixed Set in Cases of Schizopathia (1938).
36. K. D. Mdivani, The Fixed Set of Patients with Tuberculosis (1939) [jointly with Professor Kavtaradze].
37. K. D. Mdivani, "The Fixed Set in Psychasthenia" (candidate dissertation, 1946) [published in Proc. First Session, Acad. Sci. Georgian SSR, 1941].
38. K. D. Mdivani, "The Process of Extinction of the Illusions During Prolonged Exposure," Tr. Tbilissk. Gos. Univ. 18 (1940).
39. K. D. Mdivani, Weakening of the Illusion in Critical Experiments (1942).
40. A. N. Mosiava, "Experimental Material in Relation to the Problem of Objectivization," Psikhologiya 3 (1946).
41. A. N. Mosiava, "The Role of Objectivization in the Interchange of Sets," Psikhologiya 4 (1947).
42. A. N. Mosiava, Power of Objectivization in Children Seven Years Old, (1946).
43. R. G. Natadze, "Formation of a Set Based on Equality," Tr. Tbilissk. Gos. Univ. 17 (1941).
44. R. G. Natadze, The Problem of the Fixed Set Stimulated by Imagination (1945).
45. R. G. Natadze, "The Connection Between Capacity for Theatrical Representation and the Ability to Produce a Fixed Set on the Basis of Imagination," Psikhologiya 3 (1945).
46. R. G. Natadze, "The Psychological Nature of 'Faith' in Theatrical Representation of Reality," Tr. Ped. Inst. 4 (1947).
47. R. G. Natadze, "The Role of Clarity of Ideas in Stimulation of Set Formation," Psikhologiya 5 (1948).
48. R. G. Natadze, "Intention of Reality of the Object of Imagination as a Factor in Stimulation of Sets" [given at the scientific session of the Institute of Psychology on April 17, 1948].
49. V. G. Norakidze, "Sets in Subjects with Conflicts" (candidate dissertation, 1937) [published in an abbreviated form in: Collected Transactions of Batum Pedagogic Institute in 1941].
50. V. G. Norakidze, "Character of the Personality with a Fixed, Coarse, Irradiated Set" (lecture to the Sector of Psychology, Acad. Sci., Georgian SSR 1941).
51. V. G. Norakidze, "The Premorbid Personality in Psychoneuroses of War," Psikhologiya 2 (1943).
52. V. G. Norakidze, "The Character of the Personality with a Fixed, Dynamic Set," Absts. Proc. Second Session, Division of Social Sciences, Acad. Sci., Georgian SSR (1943).
53. V. G. Norakidze, "Character of the Personality with a Fixed, Coarse, Dynamic Set," Psikhologiya 3 (1945).
54. V. G. Norakidze, "The Premorbid Personality and Hysterical Reactions," Psikhologiya 5 (1948).
55. V. G. Norakidze, "Character of the Personality with a Fixed, Variable–Labile Set," Psikhologiya 4 (1947).
56. V. G. Norakidze, Character of the Personality with a Fixed, Varible–Stable Set (1944).
57. V. G. Norakidze, Changes in Character Evoked by the Situation (Concussion, Contusion, Wounds, and so on) (1945).

58. V.G. Norakidze, "The Problem of Compensation of a Defect," Absts. Proc. Second Session, Inst. Ped. Sci., Ministry of Education, Georgian SSR (1945).
59. V.G. Norakidze, "The Problem of Variability of Character," Theses Eighth Session, Batum Pedagogic Institute (1947).
60. V.G. Norakidze, "The Premorbid Personality of Schizophrenics," Theses of the Third Session, Inst. Psychol., Acad. of Sci., Georgian SSR (1948).
61. V.G. Norakidze, "Character of the Personality and the Fixed Set" (doctoral dissertation, 1948).
62. A.S. Prangishvili, "The Problem of Confidence in the Light of Objectivization," (paper presented at a conference on problems of sets, 1948).
63. D.N. Uznadze, "Impersonalia," Chveni Metsnieraba 1:1 (1923).
64. D.N. Uznadze, Fundamentals of Experimental Psychology, "The Subpsychic," Vol. 1 (1925).
65. D.N. Uznadze, "Perception and Imagination," Izv. Tbil. Univ. 6:267 (1926).
66. D.N. Uznadze, "The Fundamental Law of Interchange of Sets," Psikhologiya 9:316 (1930).
67. D.N. Uznadze, "Einstellung sumschlag als Grundlage der Kontrasttauschungen," Ninth Internat. Cong. Psychol. (1929).
68. D.N. Uznadze, "Uber die Gewichtstauschung und ihre Analoga," Psych. Forschung 14 (1931).
69. D.N. Uznadze, Sleep and Dreams (Tbilisi, 1936).
70. D.N. Uznadze, "The Theory of Posthypnotic Suggestion," Tr. Inst. of Functional Nervous Diseases, Vol. 1 (Tbilisi, 1936).
71. D.N. Uznadze, "The Psychology of the Set," Tr. Gruz. Psikhologich. Obshchestva 1 (1938).
72. D.N. Uznadze, "Untersuchungen zur Psychologie der Einstellung," Acta Psychol. 4 (1939).
73. D.N. Uznadze, General Psychology, Tbilisi, 1940, (pp. 63-94).
74. D.N. Uznadze, "Fundamental Principles of the Psychology of Sets," Tr. Tbilissk. Gos. Univ. (1941).
75. D.N. Uznadze, "The Concept of Sets in Present-Day Experimental Psychology," Absts. Proc. Third Scientific Session, Division of Social Sciences, Acad. Sci., Georgian SSR (1944).
76. D.N. Uznadze, "The Problem of Objectivization," Tr. Inst. Functional Nervous Diseases, Vol. 2 (1946).
77. D.N. Uznadze, "The Problem of Attention in the Light of the Theory of Sets," Psikhologiya 4 (1947).
78. D.N. Uznadze, "The Internal Form of Speech," Psikhologiya 4 (1947).
79. D.N. Uznadze, "The Two Levels of Mental Life," Absts. Proc. Seventh Session Inst. Psychol. (1948).
80. D.N. Uznadze, "The Problem of Objectivization," Tr. Tbilissk. Gos. Univ. (1948).
81. D.N. Uznadze, "The Problem of Development in Psychology," Absts. Proc. Eighth Session, Inst. Psychol. (1949).
82. B.I. Khachapuridze, "The Phased Character of Alternation of Sets," (collection: data on the psychology of sets, 1938).
83. B.I. Khachapuridze, "Duration of the Experimentally Produced Set" (collection: data on the psychology of sets, 1938).
84. B.I. Khachapuridze, "The Role of the Situation in Stimulation of the Set," (collection: data on the psychology of sets, 1938).
85. B.I. Khachapuridze, "Certain Conditions of the Formation and Manifestation of Sets." Introduction to the book: Didactic Materials and Games in Connection with Certain Problems in Education of the Preschool Child, Theses (1934).
86. B.I. Khachapuridze, "The Theory of the Phased Development of Sets." Tr. Tbilissk. Gos. Univ. 17 (1941).
87. B.I. Khachapuridze, "On the Nature of Changes in Sets" (candidate dissertation), Tbilisi (1938).

88. B. I. Khachapuridze, "Certain Peculiarities in the Sets of Children," Tr. Tbil. Univ. im. Stalina, Vol. XVII (1941).
89. B. I. Khachapuridze, "The Sets of the Preschool Child from the Point of View of Stability," Trans. Sector Psychol., Acad. Sci., Georgian SSR, Psikhologiya 1 (1942).
90. B. I. Khachapuridze, "Sensory Asymmetry in Experiments Concerned with Simultaneous Comparison of Sizes," Trans. Sector of Psychology, Acad. Sci., Georgian SSR, Psikhologiya 1 (1942).
91. B. I. Khachapuridze, "Sensory Asymmetry and Fixed Sets," Abst. Proc. Scientific Session, Division of Social Sciences, Acad. Sci., Georgian SSR (1943).
92. B. I. Khachapuridze, "The Ontogenetic Development of Sensory Asymmetry," Absts. Proc. First Scientific Session, Inst. Psychol., Acad. Sci., Georgian SSR (1944).
93. B. I. Khachapuridze, "The Effect of Alcohol on the Action of the Fixed Set," Trans. Inst. Psychol., Acad. Sci., Georgian SSR, Vol. 3 (1945).
94. B. I. Khachapuridze, "The Fixed Set of the Preschool Child from the Point of View of Constancy of the Type of Set" (MS, 1942).
95. B. I. Khachapuridze, "The Problem of Measurement of the Effect of the Fixed Set (Criticism of Piaget)," Absts. Proc. Scientific Session, Tbilisi Univ. (1947).
96. Z. I. Khodzhava, "Action of the Set in Conditions of Abstraction of Material," Tbilissk. Gos. Univ. 9 (1939).
97. Z. I. Khodzhava, "Psychological Accuracy in Ya. Gogebashvili's Story 'What the Cradle Could Do'," Jubilee Collection, Tbilisi State Univ. (1940).
98. Z. I. Khodzhava, "The Psychological Mechanism of Combatant Actions in War," Summary of Lecture to a Scientific Session, Acad. Sci., Georgian SSR (1941).
99. Z. I. Khodzhava, "The Factor of Shape in the Action of Sets," Tr. Tbilissk. Gos. Univ. 17 (1941).
100. Z. I. Khodzhava, "Sets and Habits," Summary of Lecture to Scientific Session, Acad. of Sci., Georgian SSR (1941).
101. Z. I. Khodzhava, "The Role of Sets in the Skill of Reading Individual Letters," Byulleten' Akad. Nauk GSSR (1942).
102. Z. I. Khodzhava, "Action of the Set on the Reading of Whole Words," Summary of Lecture to Scientific Session, Acad., Sci., Georgian SSR (1942).
103. Z. I. Khodzhava, "The Factor of the Set in Skilled Actions" (collection: psychology), Acad. Sci., Georgian SSR (1942).
104. Z. I. Khodzhava, "Sets and Practice" (collection: psychology), Acad. Sci. Georgian SSR (1942).
105. Z. I. Khodzhava, "The Psychological Basis of the Combatant Actions of War" (collection: psychology, Vol. 2, 1943).
106. Z. I. Khodzhava, "Sets and Inhibition in Reading Skill," Summary of Lecture to Session, Acad. Sci., Georgian SSR (1943).
107. Z. I. Khodzhava, "Further Experiments to Explain Inhibition of Identical Stimuli," Summary of Lecture to a Scientific Session, Acad. Sci., Georgian SSR (1942).
108. Z. I. Khodzhava, "Phonetic Dissimilation and Assimilation as a Product of the Action of Sets" (MS: Lecture to Scientific Session, Institute of Language, Acad. Sci., Georgian SSR).
109. Z. I. Khodzhava, "Intensity and Phased Character of the Action of Sets in Reading Skill" (collection: psychology, Vol. 3, 1945).
110. Z. I. Khodzhava, "Effect of Experience on Perception," Trans. Batum Pedagogic Inst., Vol. 1 (1941).
111. Z. I. Khodzhava, "Practice as a Process of Fixation of Sets," Summary of Lecture to Session, Acad. Sci., Georgian SSR (1949).
112. Z. I. Khodzhava, "The Psychological Basis of Learning," Tr. Inst. Ped. Nauk. (Tbilisi) 2 (1949).
113. Z. I. Khodzhava, "The Problem of Skill in Psychology" (doctoral dissertation).
114. N. V. Chrelashvili, "The Illusion of the Fixed Set in Hens," Psikhologiya 4 (1947).
115. N. V. Chrelashvili, Illusions of the Fixed Set in Albino Rats (1947).
116. N. V. Chrelashvili, The Nature of Delayed Reactions (1948).

117. Sh. N. Chkhartishvili, The Qualitative Character of the Illusion of the Set.
118. Sh. N. Chkhartishvili, Some Problems with the Illusion of the Set.
119. Sh. N. Chkhartishvili, Basis of the Psychology of the Set.
120. N. L. Eliava, "The Process of Extinction of a Set Fixed on an Abstract Relationship," Tr. Tbilissk. Gos. Univ. 18 (1940).
121. N. L. Eliava, "The Process of Switching of a Set and its Course" (candidate dissertation, 1946).
122. N. L. Eliava, "Switching of the Set and the Act of Objectivization," Psikhologiya 4 (1947).
123. N. L. Eliava, The Process of Switching of Sets in Cases of Schizophrenia (1948).

Basic Principles of the Theory of Set*

I. THE GENERAL THEORY OF SET

1. The Nature of Mental Activity from the Viewpoint of Modern Psychology and the Crisis in This Science

Psychology, as the science of the mind, was first formulated by Aristotle, and it must be admitted that even today it retains its Aristotelian foundations. Psychology is still limited to the investigation of the traditional concepts of mental activity — cognition, sensation, and volition. Despite differences of opinion regarding the nature of these processes, they are unquestionably the essentials of our science. Psychology deals with the problem of "consciousness," which is found exclusively in the phenomena of cognition, sensation, and volition.

This point of view is accepted without reservation, even by those who consider that mental activity includes both conscious and unconscious phenomena, those who accept the presence in psychology of the problem of the "unconscious," for example, the adherents of "psychoanalysis" (Freud and others). According to Freud, the concept of the unconscious does not imply a positive definition. It is simply the negation of the conscious state, meaning that cases may occur in which we are unaware of any conscious mental acts or experience, but nevertheless we are equally sure that some form of mental experience is in fact present. Phenomena of this type are usually called "unconscious." However, are these experiences something special, something distinct from our conscious mental experiences?

This question appears quite straightforward if we remember that the unconscious state may sometimes leave the bounds of the unconscious, in which case it appears to be a perfectly ordinary conscious mental experience.

*This chapter represents a later monograph by the author which was combined with his earlier work for the Russian edition from which this translation was taken.

Hence, from the point of view of the psychology of the unconscious, the existence of only certain mental processes can be accepted — cognition, sensation, and volition — and these may be present in either a conscious or an unconscious state. So far, psychology does not know of the existence of any other mental processes, and it is therefore restricted to their study. Starting with Aristotle, progress in psychology has consistently been the result of investigation of these states, and even in the most recent stages of its development, in the experimental investigation of mental processes, there have been no advances made beyond these usual frontiers of the investigation of the mind.

What results have been obtained from the many years of study of the phenomena of cognition, sensation, and volition? Since the beginning of the present century, it seems that everywhere voices are raised claiming that a crisis exists in our science. Questions are asked regarding the possibility of a truly scientific psychology, and suggestions are made for its renewal, either on the basis of the old position, psychology as the science of consciousness (Gestalt psychology), or on a completely new basis — the basis of refusal to study the mind and concentration of the efforts of investigators on problems of acts of behavior (behaviorism). Despite some progress in these and many other less fundamental directions, it is considered that this crisis in our science still persists even today. Bourgeois psychology is unquestionably in a blind alley, from which it cannot escape.

2. The Starting Point of Psychology is not Mental Phenomena, but the Living Individuals in Whom These Mental Phenomena Exist.

What is the reason for this state of affairs? Analysis of bourgeois psychology shows that its foundations are insecure and reforms affecting only superficial problems cannot satisfactorily resolve the problems in our science. The fact is that psychology, from the very beginning, has tried to study the processes of mental life — the processes of cognition, sensation, and will. It considers, moreover, that all these processes were given directly and initially, and that, therefore, there can be no fundamental difficulty in the method of their study, and that a detailed analysis of mental processes can lead directly to the establishment of the laws of human mental life and to the elucidation of the distinctive features of our behavior.

Bourgeois psychology, of course, cannot escape the fact of the decisive importance of personality, it cannot completely ignore the fact that the active participation in the process of vital relationships is not one of man's functions — the active participant is man himself, as an active subject. When, however, we ask what man is from the mental point of view, what we mean by his personality, traditional psychology turns to the initial concepts of mental processes and attemps to construct an idea of personality on the basis of these concepts.

Hence, personality is an arbitrary concept, deduced from the special concepts of human mental activity, but nevertheless it is proclaimed as the origin and basis of human mental life. This must probably explain the fact that the problem of personality is either disregarded in courses in psychology, or it is considered only at the end, after the phenomena of mental life have been fully discussed and the opportunity is then available for trying to reduce the concept of personality to the terms of these phenomena.

There is no doubt, however, that it is the subject himself, and not the individual acts of his mind, that takes part in his active relationships with the outside world; and if this fact is taken as the starting point, psychology, as a science, must clearly start, not with the concept of individual mental processes, but with the concept of the subject himself as a whole, who, when taking part in some form of interaction with the outside world, becomes forced to seek the help of individual mental processes. Of course, the subject himself is primary in this case and his mental activity appears as something arbitrary. Marx originally drew attention to this fact and formulated his idea as follows: "By the first method of examination [that is, in bourgeois psychology — D.U.], the starting point is consciousness [the mind — D.U.], as a living individual; by the second, which corresponds to real life, the starting point is the actual living individuals themselves, and consciousness is regarded merely as their consciousness" ("German Ideology," Partizdat TsK VKP (b), 1935, p. 17). By stressing this principle, Marx laid the foundation of the idea that it was possible to create a concrete science of psychology. However, he was unable to develop this science himself, and presented it as a task for the future.

Marx's principle clearly shows that the science of psychology, when considering the object of its investigation, starts from the concept of mental states, which are not phenomena of concrete mental activity, but which are undoubtedly abstract, radically separate from the living reality of human activity. However, the primary task of psychology is to study this activity, on the basis of which arises the whole superstructure of our mental function — our cognition, our sensation, and our volition. Having taken up this essential position, psychology must in the first place examine what this activity is, and which of its concrete elements may be revealed and investigated by our usual scientific methods. This means that our science is called upon to undertake the psychological analysis and study of the principles of human activity, insofar as this activity is the basis on which mental life grows and develops. With this interpretation of human mental activity, according to which it incorporates the activity of the subject as a whole, it is assumed that psychology must begin its work by investigating the subject, the personality as a whole, and not the individual elements of his mental activity. The study of this sphere of reality subsequently shows us that human mental activity also — the phenomena of man's consciousness, studied hitherto as to some extent independent entities — is nothing more than further specifications or definitions of the subject, definitions of this integral personality. In this case, psychology appears to us as the science of the concrete mental life of the subject, and not as the science of abstract mental phenomena, a description which can justly be applied to modern psychology in bourgeois countries.

3. The Possibility and Importance of the Study of Primary Forms of Activity in Man

If we examine the human mind from the developmental point of view, we have to recognize that our mental processes — our acts of consciousness, sensation, and volition — are no more than rigidly defined products of development, and that they can appear or develop as such only as a result of progress along the lengthy path of evolution. However, we know that the process of development is not simply a process of quantitative growth of a developing phenomenon; we know that it also includes degrees of qualitative changes. Consequently, when discussing the development of the mind, we have no reason to consider that its modern forms are the same as its ancient forms, having undergone no qualitative changes. We must accept that the mind passed along a lengthy path of changes before it was determined in its modern forms of cognition, sensation, and volition, and that it also has initial forms of manifestation, which preceded its modern forms.

Our next task is to study these forms of mental activity and, concurrently with this, to examine the question of the participation and role of these forms in the mental life of modern man.

How is this to be done? It would be most natural to turn to representatives of phylogenetically earlier stages of development of the animal kingdom and to try to examine how affairs stand with them; what is the nature of their vital activity, and do they exhibit forms of behavior governed by something other than the acts of mental life which we know in man — something other than cognitive, emotional, and volitional mental processes. However, this would not be productive. Without any idea of the primitive forms of mental life, the initial factors lying at the basis of vital activity, we should find nothing in animals, for at our stages of development they appear so strange and so inaccessible to us.

Our best course would therefore be to observe ourselves, to observe behavior at the human level of development. The data here are more extensive and, more important, they are more understandable than they would be in observations on animals, and it would be easier to detect or observe new and hitherto unreported phenomena than in animals, which we understand badly, if at all. We would find it easier to observe these new factors in our mental life, but not only to observe them, to make them also into the special object of our observation from different points of view, depending on how they appear to us in each particular case. In short, there is no doubt that the study of these phenomena at the human level of development would be more successful than at the level of development of animals so far removed from us.

The question, however, arises here: Would the study of the early stages of development of vital activity at the very high level which man occupies be of interest to us? If we remember that at higher stages of development, the preceding forms are not abolished and replaced by new forms, but are preserved, although in an abbreviated form, then clearly this question can be answered satisfactorily. The study of these early stages in man gives us an admittedly elementary, but nevertheless the clearest available, idea of all that we could otherwise obtain, and it is sufficient to allow us to make it subsequently the special object of our observation, not only in man, but in animals themselves. Obviously, therefore, our main task at present is to discover the nature of the primary forms of vital activity represented in modern man.

4. The Set as a Factor in the Integral Personality and Conditions of Its Activity

What are these early forms of behavior in man? Vital activity in its widest sense can be regarded as activity directed towards the preservation and development of the subject's life. Obviously, therefore, during the study of behavior at all levels of its development, the most fundamental role belongs to the concept of need, without which life in general would be inconceivable.

However, before this vital activity can be carried out, definite conditions are required: First, suitable food must be available in the natural surroundings. The animal must develop an active relationship to nature in order to obtain food from it. However, this can only happen if the organism is actually in need of food, if a corresponding need is present.

Hence, an interaction of active character will develop between the living organism and the environment only if some definite form of need appears in the organism, and if the environment contains the means for satisfying this need. We may say that any behavior of a living being, at whatever level it stands, unconditionally presupposes the presence of these two conditions: The presence of need and a situation for its satisfaction.

If we examine the whole complex pattern of development of the living organism as far as man, with his complex mental life, we find that behavior is based everywhere on these two basic factors. Without need and the conditions for its satisfaction, without subjective and objective factors, there can be no behavior. Undoubtedly, in the course of development of life, needs have changed considerably; new ones have appeared and old ones have sometimes become so complex that they are almost unrecognizable. However, their nature remains the same — they are still needs. Clearly, the same can be said of the means of their satisfaction; they have changed along with the needs, but they are still means for the satisfaction of needs. To sum up, the concepts of need and the situation for its satisfaction are essential concepts, without which the behavior of man or of living creatures in general would be inconceivable.

Here, however, we are concerned with the problem of the psychological nature of the relationship between need and situation, the basis of the definite character of behavior of the animal organism, in particular, that of man. For this purpose, we can utilize the accurate data obtained from our experiments. Let us take as an example a case of the expression of a definite need. Let us suppose that I feel an intense thirst and, in this state, I walk past a place where cold drinks are sold, a place which, moreover, I pass several times every day. This time however, I feel that the sight of the drinks attracts me, draws me to them. Submitting to this attraction, I stop and order a drink, the one which appears to me to be most attractive. As soon as I have quenched my thirst, the drinks lose their attraction for me, and if I pass the same place in this state, it will either be of no interest to me or I may not even notice it at all.

Attention has been drawn to this phenomenon previously (the Aufforderungscharakter of Lewin), but it has not been properly understood and utilized in science. Analysis of this universally known phenomenon, which is constantly being encountered, shows that it is a phenomenon of unusually great theoretical importance, which must receive its due place in psychology.

Hence, when I develop a certain need, the object which can satisfy it attracts me, causing me to perform an act capable of satisfying this need. In other words, if a need and a situation for its satisfaction are present, a specific state develops in the subject which may be described as a tendency, an inclination, or a state of preparation for the performance of the act capable of satisfying this need. Admittedly, this tendency is not always experienced, and then only in cases in which satisfaction is not delayed indefinitely or long enough to cause some degree of strain on the subject's powers. In ordinary cases, the matter does not proceed far enough to be reflected in the subject's emotions. This does not mean, however, that in other cases this state is not reflected in some way in the subject. We must recognize that when a need and the situation for its satisfaction are present, the subject develops a specific state which may be described as one of "preparedness," as a set toward a definite activity aimed at the satisfaction of his present need.

Hence, we may conclude that the activity of any living being, including man, may be activated in other ways than by the participation of his individual, conscious mental function, or of his cognitive, emotional, and volitional acts; it may be activated by his sets, which reflect, not his individual mental function, but the state of the subject as a whole.

If we remember that in this particular case we are dealing with the activity of the subject as a whole, then clearly activity of this type may also be accepted at other degrees of development, at which matters have not progressed as far as the appearance of specialized conscious mental functions, such as cognition, sensation, and volition. In this case, we shall be perfectly justified in stating that behavior arises much sooner than the development of our conscious functions, that the presence of mental bases of behavior must and can be determined everywhere, that we are concerned with living organisms at every state of their development. Consequently, the question naturally arises of the development of the psychological bases of behavior, the successive stages of its advance and upward movement: Psychology must consider the question of sets.

It should first be explained what is meant by sets in comparison with the ordinary experiences hitherto studied in psychology — whether sets are some special type of fact — cognitive, emotional, or volitional. Psychologists have often directed their attention to a phenomenon which they have discovered for the first time and has not previously been described, but it has always happened that this has been one of a group of special cases from the field of the main categories of conscious mental life — the field of cognition, sensation, and volition — and no one has yet made a serious attempt to cross the ordinary boundaries of the mind and to describe the presence of something fundamentally different from everything traditionally identified in it. This applies not only to the phenomena of mental activity, but also to the personality, to the subject of this activity, since the usual classes of mental life have been regarded as the elementary or primary data; and in the question of personality we have had to be content with these facts out of necessity.

Hence, the very first steps of traditional psychology, the claim that only conscious forms of mental activity exist, that there is no mind outside cognition, sensation, and volition, has led the traditionalist representatives of our science to deny in fact the existence of an integral active subject of mental life and to reduce the concept of personality to the sum total of its mental experiences.

5. Set as a Fundamental Problem in Psychology

As we have shown above, there are considerable grounds for justifying, or more accurately, for compelling the recognition of this concept of the integral subject — the concept of personality — as the starting point for the analysis of mental life. During the investigation of the living, integral man, of man himself and not of the individual element of his activity, we find that whenever a subject exhibits a need and the situation for its satisfaction is present, he develops a state of preparedness, a tendency, or, better still, a set toward a definite activity giving him satisfaction. This set is the "modus" of the subject at each concrete moment of his activity, an integral state which differs fundamentally from all his differentiated mental powers and abilities.

Turning now to the scientific study of sets, during the analysis of any behavior we must first emphasize that some form of qualitatively distinctive, specific change must take place in the state of the sets of the subject concerned. It must be remembered that in any situation during the solution of the problem, the subject first reacts as such, he reacts as a whole, but not simply as a carrier of individual psychophysical forces, to be used as material or tools for the solution of the present problems.

Obviously, therefore, the analysis of mental activity must begin with the study of the modification of the active subject as a whole, with the study of his sets.

Our original thesis, differing radically from everything on which psychology has been based, is the thesis of the falsity of the hypothesis that a direct connection exists between mental function and reality, the thesis lying at the basis of the whole psychological thought of bourgeois science. It is not the external situation or environment and the mental powers or abilities of the subject which are closely connected with and dependent on each other, as this thesis asserts, but above all the subject himself and the situation in which he solves this problem. Naturally, therefore, it is not the concept of subject or personality which must be interpreted on the basis of his individual mental powers and properties, but, on the contrary, these mental forces and properties, the individual mental functions of the subject, which must be interpreted on the basis of the subject himself. If the fundamental psychological nature of the subject is revealed to us in each case of his activity as definite modifications of his sets, this means that the fundamental and decisive problem in his psychology is the problem of sets.

6. "Perception" as a Factor in the Set: The Two Meanings of this Term

We have seen that if a need and a situation for its satisfaction are present for an animal, it develops a specific, integral state — a state of a set to a definite activity designed for the satisfaction of the present need. Is this possible, however, without the preliminary perception of an actual situation? Before a subject turns to a particular situation to use it for the satisfaction of a present need, he must have perceived this situation, he must have perceived the object capable of satisfying him. Consequently, it may be supposed that if both the need and the object, as the condition for its satisfaction, are present, a subject can perform the corresponding activity only if he perceives the presence of this object, if he makes it the object of his perception. Otherwise (we are not concerned here with the complex problem of searching), he will remain in a state of inactivity.

Hence, we must evidently recognize that if an actual need and the object capable of satisfying it are present, the subject must first notice or "perceive" this object in order that, having developed a set, he can then begin to perform the appropriate acts designed to satisfy his need. In brief, "perception" of objects determining behavior arises before the sets toward this behavior. *

On the other hand, however, we know that perception of something is a no-less complete, independent activity than any other form of behavior. The only difference lies in the greater or lesser complexity of the activity which we call behavior. In this case, naturally, the fact of perception cannot precede his set, but can only follow it. Before the subject can perform a definite, goal-directed act, in particular an act of perception, as the subject of this behavior he must first develop an integral state which can direct his activity — he must develop a set to this perception.

Hence, we see that perception must be understood, on the one hand, as the state preceding the development of the set, and, on the other hand, as an experience following this act. Is this possible?

Careful analysis shows that there are two different stages in the activity of our perceptual ability. Let us examine the first stage.

If we admit that the stimulus acts directly on our sensory organ, without the participation of personal interests and intentions, if this stimulus, without provoking the personality itself to corresponding activity, concerns only his sensory organ, then it is natural to suppose that it is not the subject, not the personality, which reacts to this stimulation but only the organ receiving the stimulus. Clearly, in this case the subject's set remains unaffected, outside the influence of the stimulus which is affecting not the subject himself, but one of the organs of his body. This can take place most easily if the subject is uninterested in his surroundings; if, as a

*See Editor's note 3.

subject or personality, he is completely excluded from the chain of events unfolding around him. This can happen, for example, when we are asleep. During sleep, the whole practical association between a living organism and the environment ceases completely; sleep involves the exclusion of all active links with the surrounding reality.

When we wake up, however, as a result of the action of some external impressions, for example, a strong acoustic stimulus, before we are wide awake and are still, as it were, on the way toward awakening, we do not feel this impression as something acting upon us from outside. We feel it rather as a state of our organ of hearing, as a noise in our ears, but not as a sound proceeding from the surrounding world, for instance, the sound of a rough sea.

This state, it must be supposed, is found not only during awakening from sleep. It is, in general, characteristic of living beings, and, in particular, of man, and all forms of perception begin with a state of this type. Admittedly, we usually do not notice it, but this is only because the subject quickly develops a practical relationship with reality and, in particular, with all the impressions acting upon him from the outside world.

Hence, we may conclude that the stage of development of the set, as a state of a subject or personality, is preceded by a primary effect of the action of a stimulus on one of his sensory organs — an effect which cannot yet be regarded as a true, complete perception of a definite, objective stimulus, localized in the outside world. It would therefore be most natural to describe this stage of perception as the stage of "noticing" or, more exactly, the stage of "sensation" of stimuli acting from outside.

Before true perception can be obtained, the intervention of the subject is required, the participation of his set in a definite form. If the presence of a need, a situation for its satisfaction, and the sensation of stimuli acting on this situation can be accepted, it can readily be concluded that in these conditions the subject must initiate his activity as an integral, living organism and that, consequently, in order to do this he must first develop a set corresponding to this activity — he must develop a set toward the perception in which he is interested.

The perception obtained on this basis — true, complete perception — must be regarded as the next stage in the development of the perceptual power of the living being. This second stage of development of perception, the stage which in man is subsequently followed by the third stage, is the stage of objectivization, which we shall discuss below when studying the specific features of the set.

To conclude our analysis of the conditions of development of the set, we must examine from a different point of view the concept of this preliminary "noticing" or "sensation," preceding the development of the set. What does it mean?

We know that the mind is not something new and independent of matter. On the contrary, it must be conceived as a property appearing at a definite stage of development of matter. Admittedly, in a clearly defined form, the mind is linked in the form of sensation only with the higher forms of matter, but this does not mean that earlier forms of the mind may exist, preceding sensation, as the "clearly defined form" of its development. Lenin declares that "At the foundations of the edifice of matter, we can only postulate the existence of a faculty similar to sensation" (V. I. Lenin, "Materialism and Empiriocriticism," Partizdat TsK VKP(b), 1936, p. 30). Clearly, therefore, the mind (in this case, sensation) has an historial background, its more primitive forms must be supposed to be hardly "at the foundation of the edifice of matter," and the more highly developed mental processes (for example, sensation) are preceded at various stages of development of matter by corresponding stages of the development of "sensation" (mental).

However, if this is so, if mental properties in general appear during the process of development and not during the development of matter, in this case it is undoubtedly true that sensation and, still more, perception passed through a series of stages of development — that there is no such thing as a single perception, representing all the possible forms of its development, but that on the contrary, it is more correct to consider that there are different stages of perception which should be differentiated from each other.

It can therefore be concluded that different stages of development of perception exist. Without investigating the problem of the development of these stages, we may nevertheless consider that one of its possible lines of development must have been in the direction of growth of the independence of this function. Perception has acquired a comparatively independent value in the processes of cognition, and at its high levels of development it has become a completely independent mental act. Cases are known in which a person has had to carry out a series of observations on a certain concrete fact, as a completely independent task, in order subsequently to find a place for it in the system of analogous phenomena.

It will be noted that the stages passed through earlier do not disappear on the appearance of new and more advanced stages of development. They continue to exist side by side, although in a contracted form.

Hence, the basic principle of the theory of behavior can be summarized as follows: For any phenomenon of behavior to appear, it must be assumed that a living being, with the ability of primitive perception and some form of activated need capable of being satisfied in these environmental conditions, develops a relationship with this environment on the basis of the integral state of the set arising in the subject, which leads him to perform purposive actions.

7. Diffuse, Differentiated, and Fixed Sets

We will now turn to the question of the course of human activity. We have previously shown that the onset of activity is directly preceded by a set, an integral state of the active personality, and the whole of his activity subsequently takes place under the controlling influence of this set. The activity of the personality in connection with the solution of a particular problem is essentially nothing more than the putting into operation of his set. Let us examine the course of this process. We may assume that we have a subject in whom, for the first time, a need has arisen in conditions capable of satisfying this need. We know that in such a situation, the subject must develop a set toward a particular type of activity, capable of bringing him satisfaction. Let us assume that in this case the subject's experience plays no part and he has to solve the problem facing him for the first time in his life. What happens in this case? It is easy to imagine that the subject in these conditions may not consider the situation for his activity specifically enough; that is, he may not be able to develop the necessary activity in accordance with all the conditions of the external environment necessary for the successful solution of the problem. The set appearing in this case is not the state of a subject capable of accurately satisfying his need, but instead it is characterized by a certain vagueness or diffuseness, requiring further action on the part of the specific conditions of solution of the problem before it can become a definitive state of the subject, directing his activity along the lines appropriate to this situation.

Hence, we must realize that during the early stage of action of a situation on a subject, as a rule the sets are diffuse.

This forces us to consider the measures to be taken to produce further differentiation of sets, and the only method available in this case is the organization of the repeated action of the particular condition for satisfaction of the need on the subject. We may expect that, as a result of this repeated action of the situation, the subject elaborates and differentiates the appropriate set, and as such it becomes fixed. In this way, our subject develops a fixed set with a certain degree of differentiation.

8. Experiments with Fixed Sets

In the normal condition of life, the most characteristic form of set is the differentiated set, which, as a rule, is at the same time a fixed set. Because of this fact, we can make a more detailed, comprehensive study of the set, for we have been presented with wide opportunities for the experimental analysis of the facts relating to the activity of the set. We may ask a subject, in whom we first create a need to solve an experimental problem, to say, for example, which of two objects given to him appears to be larger (usually in these experiments, the subject is given two balls differing from each other considerably in size). The presentation of these objects is repeated several (10 to 15) times so that the set which arises in each individual case (the set on the assessment "bigger" or "smaller") becomes adequately fixed. Next, assuming that the subject has a fixed set—assessment of the size of two objects of different sizes (in this case, two wooden balls)—at the next presentation (the eleventh to sixteenth), we replace the ordinary balls, which were used to fix his set, by two of the same size, and we ask him to say which is which (this experiment will reveal the presence of a fixed set in our subject, so that we call it the critical experiment). We consider that if a subject actually develops a set and it is fixed in the course of repeated presentations, when he is shown balls of equal size, he will perceive them as unequal, as a result of the fixation of the set during the preceding presentation, which we call fixing exposures.

9. Experiments on the Integral, Personal Nature of the Set

These experiments enable us to make an experimental study of the set, at least in its fixed form, and we use them here first to solve the cardinal problem of the integral, personal character of the set.

Let us first consider the problem that the set in man precedes his conscious mental processes, that it is a fact from the sphere of human activity which has hitherto been called the sphere of the unconscious mind.

Let us carry out fixing experiments in our subjects, but in a specific state — in the state of hypnotic sleep. This means that, after a subject has fallen asleep under the influence of hypnotic suggestion, balls of different sizes are placed successively into his hands 10 to 15 times and then, having been instructed to forget all about these experiments, he is taken into another room, where he is brought out of his hypnotic state. Having asked him what happened to him while he was asleep, and being satisfied that the subject remembers nothing of the experiments carried out with him, the experimenter then places balls of the same size into his hands (critical objects) and asks him to compare them.

These experiments, carried out with a series of different persons, as a rule gave the same result: The balls used as critical objects were identified as unequal; one ball appeared much bigger than the other, and in the same order as they appeared to be unequal to the subjects in the ordinary, and not the hypnotic, fixing experiments.

What can we learn of this result of our hypnotic experiments? Clearly, the equal balls of the critical experiments appeared unequal to the subjects only because of the preceding fixing experiments. This means that the effect of these experiments persisted completely; that is, in the fixing experiments the subjects developed a set which left no trace in their consciousness — they remembered absolutely nothing about these experiments. Nevertheless, this set persisted outside their consciousness, and in the critical experiments it exerted its appropriate influence on the perception of the equal balls. The balls appeared obviously unequal to the subjects, under the definite influence of the fixing experiments, although let us repeat, they remembered absolutely nothing about their results.

Consequently, we must conclude that, in accordance with these experiments, the subject develops a set which, since he knows nothing about its existence, cannot be a part of his consciousness or, what amounts to the same thing, it cannot be considered a special mental fact; undoubtedly, this set must be regarded as a state of the subject as a whole. This, then, is the result of the facts of posthypnotic suggestion.

Consequently, the set is a state of the personality, its modus at each particular moment, but it is not one of its special mental functions, having a local distribution and a corresponding importance.

The subject is successively given, for example, a pair of balls into his right hand — at first a bigger one, followed by a smaller. This is repeated 10 to 15 times (fixing experiments). These are followed by the critical experiments: Into the subject's other hand (in this case, the left) is placed a pair of balls of the same size. As a rule, one of these balls (the first) appears bigger than the second. Consequently, an illusion of volume is also obtained in the hand which took no part in the fixing experiment, and if, as a result of these, a set to "the first ball is bigger" was produced, it was of course produced in the hand taking part in the fixing experiments. But this was the right hand, not the left. Nevertheless, an illusion was actually obtained in this hand. What does this mean? The only conclusion which can be drawn in this case is as follows: The fixing experiments carried out with the right hand were sufficient to produce a set not only in this hand, but also in the left, that is, in the corresponding organ.

Consequently, fixing experiments in one hand create a set not only in left hand, but also in the other, taking no part in the experiment. Clearly, sets fixed in the region of one hand also spread to the other hand.

We may repeat the same experiment in the sphere of vision. Fixing experiments are carried out with one eye (let us say, the right), and critical experiments with the other eye. The results obtained are similar to those of the preceding experiments; that is, with the left eye we perceive equal objects as unequal. The first appears smaller than the second — we have here the ordinary illusion of the set. A set arising in relation to the right eye automatically spreads to the left.

Now let us carry out fixing experiments with the hands and critical experiments in the optic region; that is, we will place a larger ball into the right hand and a smaller ball into the left hand. We shall carry out the critical experiment in the optic sphere; that is, we shall show the subject two balls of different sizes so that he may compare them and state how they are related in size.

The results in this case also show that a set, if produced haptically, also acts in the optic sphere. Corresponding experiments show that the same applies if the relationship between the fixing and critical experiments is reversed; a set produced in the optic sphere also acts in the haptic sphere.

To sum up, we can conclude that a set fixed in one sensory modality is at the same time fixed in all other modalities.

What do these results show? There can be only one answer. The set is evidently not a phenomenon of a special order, and it cannot be interpreted as a state of one particular organ; it is not a phenomenon of local character but, on the contrary, it extends to all our organs of perception; it is a state of the organism as a whole — the whole subject as such.

We may conclude that the set is not a special mental phenomenon among a series of other similar phenomena, but something integral, characterizing the state of the subject's personality.

Hence, all these experiments show that sets do not belong to the ordinary categories of mental phenomena — the categories of cognition, sensation, and volition, but that, on the contrary, having no special or local character, they must be regarded as falling into the integral, personal category.

10. The Problem of the Unconscious

Philosophical thought has long been concerned with the presence of phenomena in the human mind which it has called "unconscious." This concept plays a particularly important role in the theory of psychoanalysis. Freud considers that man's mental life is largely based on processes taking place in the region of the unconscious. He has developed a whole system of ideas relating to the problem of the unconscious mind. However, as we have mentioned above, Freud's concept of the unconscious has introduced nothing new which is not found in the phenomena of the conscious mind. He describes as unconscious an experience which we have sometimes recognized as a definite mental phenomenon, as a definite desire or thought, and which in the future may be revealed to us in the form of similar definite facts of mental life. According to Freud, the practical purpose of psychoanalysis is that it helps the subject to draw the curtains from his unconscious experiences and to show them in their true form, that is, to make them into ordinary conscious mental facts.

Freud's view of the nature of the unconscious is undoubtedly fundamentally incorrect. Having based his system on this concept, when describing it he is compelled to use mainly a negative concept, declaring simply that there are certain facts which possess the quality of consciousness, but if lacking in this quality they must therefore be called unconscious. So far as their positive characteristics are concerned, they have none (according to Freud), and for this reason he has no choice but to call them unconscious. But here is a strange thing! With this purely negative understanding of the unconscious, in practice Freud has frequently achieved positive results in the treatment of psychoses. It would be facile to deny that such results have been obtained — they unquestionably have. On the other hand, however, it is equally unquestionable that the theory of the unconscious mind, as Freud understands it, has given no positive contribution to science, and it is clearly impossible, therefore, that this theory should be responsible for the actual success obtained in the treatment of these patients. It must be assumed that, in the course of treatment, Freud frequently succeeded in influencing what was largely responsible for the disease — the factor which he could define only negatively as unconscious. However, he did not see the positive side of this concept, a fact to which can be attributed all the extremes of his theory.

We concluded above that, besides the ordinary mental factors, besides individual conscious mental experiences, we must accept the presence of a modus of the state of the subject receiving these experiences, a set of his personality. Obviously, the integral state is not reflected in the subject's consciousness as individual independent experiences — its role is to determine the subject's work in a direction of activity leading him to the satisfaction of his needs. This state of the subject as a whole cannot be experienced by him as a series of individual facts characterizing the situation in which his activity takes place.

A set cannot be an individual act in a subject's consciousness, but only a modus of his state as a whole. It may naturally be considered, therefore, that if something in us takes place unconsciously, it must of course be our set.

Hence, we see that the unconscious actually exists in us, but that this unconscious is none other than the subject's set.

Consequently, the concept of unconscious from this moment ceases to be a purely negative concept, but acquires a fully positive significance and must be analyzed in science on the basis of ordinary methods of investigation.

11. Further Characteristics of the Set

Special investigations of the set have shown that this concept has a general character — it concerns both phenomena of quantitative relationships and phenomena of qualitative differences — and methods exist for the study of all these, making them accessible to experimental analysis. However, we shall not discuss this problem in particular, like many other problems concerned with the general aspects of the set. We shall simply note a few conclusions drawn from investigations of problems of the set of a general character.*

We can now give a more or less detailed definition of the set in relation to the following aspects: (1) the aspect of the varieties of sets, (2) the aspect of excitability of the set, (3) the aspect of its extinction, and (4) the aspect of its extinction in the conditions of prolonged exposures and when it follows a natural course.

From the results of our experiments, we can now distinguish between a diffuse, an undifferentiated, and a fixed set; we can distinguish between a readily excitable set, undergoing fixation after a few fixing experiments, and an unfixable set, excitable with difficulty or not at all; furthermore, as a result of experiments on the extinction of the set, several varieties may be distinguished, and their properties are fully defined in this series of experiments: (1) a dynamic set, disappearing after a series of repeated critical experiments, and a static set, which does not disappear in the course of this series of experiments; (2) a plastic set, gradually becoming weaker and giving place to a new set, corresponding to the current experimental situation only after passing through a series of stages, and a coarse set which is extinguished immediately. without passing through this series of stages of extinction.

It is also important to mention that the set usually passes through stages of extinction regardless of how the critical experiments are given: whether as usual, that is, successive exposures of critical objects, or the prolonged action of these objects on the subject until the complete disappearance of the illusion arising on the basis of the fixed set. In both cases, the results are the same: At first an illusion of contrast develops, followed by an assimilative illusion, and, finally, the subject states that the critical objects are equal.

Finally, if the critical experiments are carried out, not immediately after the fixing experiments, but after a variable interval of time (hours, days, months), it can be seen that fixed sets may exist in more or less labile (the set disappears soon) or stable (the set remains active for a long time) forms.

*D. N. Uznadze, "The Experimental Basis of the Psychology of Sets," Psikhologiya 6 (1949).

Various other problems are considered in the general theory of sets, such as, for example, the question of sets based on equality, sets based on qualitatively identical phenomena, and so on; but at present we are doing no more than giving a brief account of the general theory of sets, which is essential for the understanding of the subsequent text.

Our next purpose must be to examine the problem of sets at different stages of their phylogenetic development — sets in animals and in man.

II. THE PROBLEM OF SET IN ANIMALS

1. The Problem of Set in Animals and the Method of Investigation

As we have seen above, the essential conditions for the development of a set are so elementary that there is no question that they may exist even at low levels of development of the animal world. In fact, however elementary the structure of a living organism, it has definite needs which are satisfied in suitable environmental conditions. Like these two fundamental conditions for the activity of a set, the third is also elementary — a primitive level of perception, essential for the development of any set. Consequently, all three conditions necessary for the appearance of a set are present in animals.

In order to prove that sets in fact exist in animals, the best course is to make an experimental analysis of this problem.

Of all the possible experiments, we shall discuss those which are basically the same as those carried out with human subjects. Of course, they must be simplified sufficiently to make them suitable for animals.

As an example, we shall describe briefly one experimental method used to investigate sets in animals. The basic requirement which must be satisfied by this technique is as follows: It must activate a need in the animal which can serve as the basis for its activity directed toward the solution of a problem. In man, this is done by the use of a spoken message, but in animals this is impossible, so the experiment must be so devised that its conditions directly activate the need impelling the animal to turn to behavior directed toward its satisfaction. Otherwise, the method includes nothing specific other than, of course, the general experimental conditions which must be so devised as to take account of the special features of the behavior of the animals used as subjects in each individual case. For example, a hen is shown two surfaces on which grain is scattered. On one surface, namely, the dark surface, the grain can be pecked freely, while on the other, the lighter surface, this cannot be done because the grain has been glued to the surface. In the fixing experiments, the hen becomes accustomed to pecking from the comparatively dark surface, and ultimately it no longer pecks from the light surface. Hence, by means of an adequate number of fixing experiments, the set to peck from the darker surface becomes fixed in the bird. In critical experiments, the hen is shown two surfaces, one of which is colored the same as the lighter fixing background (b), to which it was accustomed not to react, while the other (c) is lighter still. As might have been expected, the hen pecked from surface b, despite the fact that in the fixing experiment it did not react at all to a surface of this color.

We may conclude from these normal reactions of the hen that in these experimental conditions, analogous with Köhler's well-known experiments, the set to peck from the darker background becomes fixed in the bird. It seems to us that this explanation of the reaction of the hen in these experiments is much simpler than any other.

Our other fixing experiments with animals showed conclusively that a set may become activated and that their activity will be determined by this set.*

At the present time, as a result of an extensive series of experiments with other animals (albino rats, monkeys, dogs), it is well established that sets may also be based on the activity of animals and that they may easily be subjected to experimental analysis, like the sets in experiments with human subjects.

2. Distinctive Features of Sets in Animals

What can we say about sets in animals?

First, it has been found that sets may arise not only in full agreement with everything we have said above concerning the appearance of sets in general, but also that they follow fundamentally the same pattern as in man. They pass through the same stages of extinction, that is, stages of contrast, assimilation and, finally, equality, and they occur in the same types (dynamic and static sets, plastic and coarse) the same forms (diffuse and differentiated sets), and the same degrees of excitability, and so on.

*See Editor's note.

However, corresponding to the comparatively low level of development of animals, all these properties of the set assume distinctive features. The first feature to draw attention is the considerable diffuseness of sets in animals. Where in man, as a rule, a well-defined, fixed, differentiated set appears, in animals it lacks this definition and appears much more often than in man as a diffuse set.

Next, as a rule sets in animals are much more variable than in man. Whereas in man they are constant in character (that is, however they are produced they always follow the same type of course), in animals, on the other hand, they may change their type and thus exhibit variability.

Finally, sets in animals, being more diffuse than in man, show some degree of specificity in their course. Whereas the fixed set in man is manifested from the beginning as one of contrast, and its assimilative form only develops later as the set becomes weaker, in animals things are rather different. Often, nearly always, it happens that the fixed set in animals is manifested from the very beginning in the form of an assimilative illusion, and the illusion of contrast begins to appear only later. Since this order of replacement of the illusions is seen far more often in animals than in man, it may be regarded as a characteristic feature of the animal set.

This fact is associated with the difficulty experienced in the fixation or excitation of sets in animals. We know that the excitability of a set can be measured by the number of fixing experiments given to the subject. As a result of experiments with animals, it was discovered that the fixation of sets in these subjects requires many more fixing experiments than in man, and even then adequate fixation of the set is not always secured.

One further feature of the set in animals merits our attention. We know from experiments with human subjects that their sets are distinguished by a varying degree of stability (that is, once fixed, they remain active for a long time); it has also been observed that, while they always remain in a fixed state, they often begin to change their type — they may gradually weaken and, eventually, they disappear completely as a rule. The situation is rather different with respect to the stability of set in animals; often it is not present at all, or if it is, the set remains active for a long time, constantly maintaining its original type; the animal continues in the power of this set for a comparatively long period.

3. The Problem of Mental Processes, Especially the Problem of Thinking in Animals

Of the many distinctive manifestations of sets in animals, we shall content ourselves with the analysis of only one. In our opinion, this is the most characteristic, or even specific, feature of the life of the set, and its analysis will help us to understand not only the animal, but also, and more important man.

We have seen that in the presence of a particular need and the conditions for its satisfaction, an animal develops a set toward appropriate activity which, as a rule, it tries to carry out. When feeling thirsty, that is, having the need to drink, the animal, if water is present, runs to it to satisfy its needs. It behaves in a similar way when other needs are dominant. For a particular form of activity to develop, aimed at the concrete satisfaction of a particular need, it is therefore necessary that the means of satisfaction of this need should be present. So long as the animal is unaware of this means, it cannot develop a set toward individual goal-directed activity. A set of this type can develop in the animal only in the presence, not only of a need, but also of a definite means of its satisfaction. A set toward concrete activity may appear as a living force only if concrete conditions for the satisfaction of this individually determined need are also present. Consequently, we may say more accurately that a set toward definite behavior appears in an animal in the presence, not only of an actual need, but also of environmental conditions essential for its satisfaction. If we examine any case of activity of an animal, we can see that it arises and develops in all cases only on the basis of these conditions.

What, then, can we say with respect to certain other psychological conditions of behavior which, in this particular case, have been completely ignored. If we are sure that in order to perform an act of behavior, an animal has only to develop and put into operation a corresponding set, in this case it will have to be accepted that, of all the mental processes, it need have only those which play the role of essential conditions for the development of its set. We have seen that this role can be played only by mental processes from which, consequently, at a higher level of development, those individual acts develop which are known in man as perception. We have shown above that these mental processes must be understood as sensation, the organs of which are also represented at the lower levels of development of the animal world.

So far as the other, more complex, mental processes are concerned, careful analysis shows that they are unnecessary for the work of an animal in the ordinary conditions of life; the animal does not utilize them, and perhaps they are absent altogether.

In that case, we must turn next to the problem of thinking in animals. This subject is a matter of particular interest at the present time. Attempts are being made to show that thinking is not entirely alien to animals, and cases in which it appears and the forms which its activity takes in animals at different levels of phylogenetic development are being studied.

Observations have shown that in experimental conditions of investigation an animal presents facts which could be interpreted as representing the activity of its intellectual faculties. However, such facts are found only when the animal is forced to act in special experimental conditions created by the investigator, that is, in conditions which have been constructed so as to guarantee success for the animal only if it carried out the activity envisaged by these conditions. However, the natural conditions of the animal's life, in which it has to face and solve problems, differ considerably and essentially from the experimental conditions in which we have compelled it to act. Clearly, therefore, our experimental animal, which shows itself capable of thinking in the experiments, may never do so in its ordinary conditions of life, for example, in the case of a monkey in the forest. The conditions of an animal's life are evidently not something abstract, which can be detached from the internal possibilities of its activity and replaced by any other conditions. The internal and external conditions of life are naturally interconnected, and before we can in fact understand an animal, we must study it in the natural conditions of its life. But in these conditions we do not know the facts which would compel us to accept in animals the presence of the processes which we know in man as processes of thought.

Hence, in animals in the natural conditions of their existence thinking does not occur. We shall see below that thought can be a regulating factor in life only in man, and that only man is an intellectual being. If, however, we must recognize that animals as such do not require thought in the natural conditions of their life, and that consequently thought does not occur, it becomes quite clear that other mental functions related in their usual activity with the work of the intellect, also may be absent from animals. For example, the function of perception, in its true meaning, assumes not only the presence of a function, but also the idea of its object; the same can be said of attention, as we shall see in particular below, and also of memory, which incorporates the idea of what is remembered. Even more is this true of volition, of the ability to realize a conscious purpose, which is only possible on the basis of thought.

Hence, in animals there can be none of those mental functions which we know to be acts presupposing an object and, consequently, closely related with thought, which in fact is absent at this level.

4. Specific Features of the Mind of the Animal: Absence of the Idea of Identity

This demonstrates to us a specific feature of the animal mind, of the utmost importance to the understanding of its entire behavior, a behavior so completely different from everything that we know in respect of specifically human activities.

The fundamental condition of any thought is the ability to recognize identity. In order to think of something, in order to predicate something, we have to assume that this something has been given to us. Thinking is the ability to predicate or, what amounts to the same thing, the ability to judge. In a nutshell, ability to perform acts of thought presupposes the preliminary possession of the idea of identity, the ability to identify.

What does this mean? It means that where there is no thought, there can be no idea of identity of anything, there can be no idea of identifying something with itself, and absolutely no idea of repetition, because this idea can occur only if there is the ability to notice and to recognize that a particular phenomenon is exactly the same phenomenon as took place before.

Hence, in the animal world the ability of identification of phenomena, the ability to see and to recognize them repeatedly, is absent.

But if this is so, if the animal is unable to experience or to notice repetition, this means that any situation which it uses to satisfy its need and any phenomenon from this situation must appear to the animal as something new or, more correctly, it must experience it in the same way without applying the attribute of new or old. Any situation must be experienced without the possibility of defining it from the point of view of repetition.

Does this mean, however, that there is no difference between old and new in an animal's behavior, that both these acts of behavior follow an identical course regardless of whether they are happening for the first time or are being repeated?

There is no doubt that repetition plays an important role in the life of an animal. For example, if it cannot obtain food by a direct method, it will try to obtain it again by the same method or, in an extreme case, by some new method. An animal frequently has to repeat its acts of behavior in order to live. This means that it is capable of identifying phenomena and objects, that it is capable of recognizing their identity. Consequently, it seems that our conclusion regarding the absence of the power of identification in animals, their unfamiliarity with the logical law of identity, is not justified.

A particularly questionable feature is the presence of this ability in animals during experiments to investigate their conditioned reflexes. We know that conditioned reflexes are produced and consolidated by the repeated application of appropriate stimuli. If the same stimulus is reinforced repeatedly for a sufficient number of times, a definite response of the animal is produced, in the form of a definite conditioned reflex. But does this mean that the animal recognizes this as repetition, and that consequently it can recognize that objects are the same, and recognize their identity?

Certainly not! The theory of conditioned reflexes shows that during the repeated application of definite stimuli, these reflexes are produced completely objectively, without the influence of subjective experiences. Repetition reproduces a definite and completely objective effect, in this case the secretion of saliva, a process which is not under conscious control, but a purely physiological fact. It is quite clear that this definite effect is produced not by the awareness of repetition, but merely by the fact of its presence. It would therefore be most suitable in this case not to mention repetition at all, because only someone capable of abstracting from the direct practical significance of active impressions and capable of studying only their interrelationships can judge that in this particular case we are in fact concerned with repetition. In any event, this can not be done by an animal.

It is therefore clear that a series of motor responses may be produced in animals by the repeated application of stimuli, but it is also clear that these responses can be explained on the basis of purely physiological processes taking place in the organism not necessarily with the participation of consciousness. It can therefore be concluded that there is no conscious repetition in animals and that, consequently, there are no grounds for assuming that animals are conscious of the identity of events taking place before them.

Obviously, therefore, the animal world cannot recognize something as equal to itself, something identical with itself. Where everything is in motion, where everything changes, there can be no repetition. With this interpretation of animal life, it is clear that the animal's mind can contain nothing whose presence could not be justified by the conditions of its existence in a world in which nothing was ever repeated; it contains no processes of thought or acts of volition, nothing from our own mental activity which would to some extent presuppose the presence of these two specifically human psychological facts.

5. The Problem of Instinct

If this is true, however, the question arises of the real possibility of various cases of behavior in animals, the presence of which it is difficult to justify in the conditions of the eternally moving, never repeating, world in which they live and act, such as the possibility of instinct. Let us examine this problem for a while, confining ourselves to a short review of the direction in which the problem of instincts may be satisfactorily solved.

Instinctive activity resembles in its character those varieties of complex activity whose appearance and course usually require the obvious participation of consciousness. However, this is not true of instincts; they arise and proceed without any participation of consciousness. When we ask what regulates this complex type of activity, remembering that there is no reason to suspect the participation of conscious regulation, we conclude that this is a distinctive type of unconscious activity which, in contrast to other forms of unconscious activity, we call instinctive. However, because of the far too obviously arbitrary character of this method of solution of the problem, the theory of instinct has never been satisfactorily enunciated. It has always aroused fresh doubts, calling for new theoretical investigation.

The problem of instinct is directly dependent on the general problem of the understanding of animal activity as a whole. Since, in its attempts to understand animal activity, animal psychology has adopted largely the principles governing human activity, it has been forced to adopt the ordinary theory of instinct which we have just mentioned. If it refused to accept these principles, it would be compelled essentially to abandon the idea that instinctive acts are in any way peculiar, and it would try to identify them with reflexes, regarding them as complex "chain" reflexes.

If, however, we begin from the concept of sets, we can begin to understand the whole of animal behavior in a completely new light. We can see that the need and the conditions of its satisfaction are never phenomena bearing a chance relationship to each other. The set of activity, arising on its basis, demonstrates the internal connection between this activity and the need which it must satisfy. This means that any animal activity, taking place on the basis of a set, is essentially purposive in character. From this point of view, the behavioral acts of an animal are indistinguishable from one another — they are all internally determined, goal-directed acts.

This is true of the whole behavior of the animal. Consequently, it cannot be held that instinctive activity differs in some essential respect from other activities. All these activities are purposive and consist of a more or less complex series of actions, a definite system, directed toward the satisfaction of the animal's current goals. The individual actions forming part of this system are not the result of conscious selection. They are all determined by the nature of the set which they are putting into practice, and there is no significant difference between them. Such instinctive actions are not essentially different from other concrete cases of activity to which the animal turns when solving problems confronting it. The problem of instinct must and can be solved only from the point of view that it is the purposive activity of an animal, aimed at the solution of a problem arising in the concrete conditions of its activity.

Hence, we can see that instinct is not a special problem and that the whole activity of an animal, irrespective of the complexity of its composition, is mainly regulated on the basis of its sets, expressing the relationship between the objective conditions of the situation and the need which they are intended to satisfy.

III. SET IN MAN

1. The Specific Conditions of Set in Man

A set is the state of a subject which changes depending on the problems which he faces and the conditions in which he solves them. This subject may be an animal, but he may also be a man, for the life of both can be reduced to the process of solution of the problems of which it consists.

However, human life differs radically from the life of the animal. Whereas the life of an animal is entirely a biological fact, the life of a man is basically something more complex; it is a socially determined process. It is therefore quite natural that the principles governing life in these two cases are not identical — the fact that human life is socially determined exerts a decisive influence on its specific course, on the principles corresponding to its more complex nature.

What are these specific features of man's behavior brought about by these events in his life? We have seen that in the animal the fundamental fact giving its whole activity its psychological direction arises on the basis of needs and the conditions of their satisfaction. Since man also is fundamentally a living being, there is no question about the necessity for satisfaction of his biological needs. Needs and situations for their satisfaction in this case also play the same role as in animals, and the sets arising on their basis are still the feature directly governing and controlling human activity.

However, everything has changed considerably in this case. In the first place, the needs themselves have changed; new needs have been born, differing considerably from the old, and this "generation of new needs is the first historical task"* of man, which continues without interruption so long as man remains an historical being. Because of this, of course, the situations in which these needs are satisfied also change. It is obvious that the subject of these needs — man — having become an historial being, also has not remained unchanged; exposed continually to the process of growth and development, he himself has become to a large extent different.

Let us first consider the most radical change in the activity of the set in man, a change which may be regarded as qualitative in character, after which we will examine some of the less important aspects of this change.

2. The Fact of Consciousness in Man

When performing some activity, an animal does so because it is forced to seek means of satisfying its immediate needs. The set which develops in this case is a set based on the satisfaction

*K. Marx and F. Engels," German Ideology," p. 18.

of these actual needs, for at that moment it has no other needs whatever. This is clear because the life of an animal is confined by the limits of the constantly changing, ceaselessly moving present.

It is a different matter with man. He sees himself as an active participant in this world of reality which he contrasts to himself as something outside him and something to which he responds in a definite manner. Not only is he a directly active principal, but at the same time he is also something that is aware of the existence of a world outside him. The animal lives and acts in this world, but is not at the same time aware of the existence of itself and of the world outside it. Man is a conscious being, and this is not true of the animal. If we approach man from the point of view of the distinctive features of his mind, we can see that the main difference between the mind of the animal and the mind of man is as follows: The animal is only an animal, it lives and acts and nothing more, whereas man not only lives and acts, but at the same time he knows what it is that lives and acts in this world existing outside him.

Such, in fact, is the difference between man and animals. We are now confronted with the special psychological problem of demonstrating the changes in the human mind responsible for such a fundamental difference between it and the mind of animals. We must demonstrate the structure of the psychological mechanism enabling man not only to act in this world, but also to see that both exist — both this world, and man himself in it.

3. Delays (Pauses in Mental Activity) as a Specifically Human Act

In order to understand this, we must make observations on certain specific cases in our lives, best of all cases in which we are in what appears to be a transitional stage. This is observed in its simplest form at the moment of waking, that is, at the moment of transition from sleep to a waking state. Suppose I hear the clock chiming in the room where I am asleep. The chimes awaken me and I hear them. However, now I am awake, and at once I feel the desire to know what the time is. It seems that in my consciousness I again hear the same chimes of the clock repeated, the chimes in fact which awakened me: I seem to hear them again clearly enough to count them, and thus to be able to tell the time. The very fact of making this observation is sufficient to show that the chimes of the clock in this case apparently occur twice — they are apparently repeated.

As a result of this case and many others like it, we can draw conclusions concerning the specific feature of the course of our waking mental life. We can see that in fact our mental processes — in this case the acts of reflection upon the chimes of the clock in our mind — take place in a time sequence, one after the other. If, however, we are able to check them, it seems that the clock chimes a second time, and we can actually count the chimes.

What is the nature of the course of mental life in ordinary conditions, when a subject has no problem currently requiring a responsible attitude toward the outside world, when he does not feel the need, not only to experience, but also to give an account of what he experiences? The observation we have just described shows that in these cases it is quite sufficient if some form of activity is taking place in our minds, and nothing more. But if we assume something completely different, namely, that our experience itself is for some reason or other a matter of independent interest for us, then the situation changes radically. In this case, I must hold on to my experience a little, check its course, and make it the subject of my observation. In brief, I must do something in order to repeat my experience, so that I can examine it and say something about it.

What does this last case represent? This is a problem of considerable interest. We have seen that the life of an animal is a process completely devoid of any such problems. But in man it is completely different! We can say that the whole of human life, in its specifically human aspect, is filled with cases of checks of this type, repetitions carried out for the purpose of examining and observing what has been halted, what has been repeated. This is an exceptionally interesting point in the difference between human and animal life. Let us examine the specific features of this process and try to analyze it as best we can.

We have said that in case of necessity, man checks his activity and, instead of continuing it, halts it at the point of interest and makes it the object of his observation. Traditional science, like everyday observation, has long stressed this fact and noted it as an obvious case of the activity of our attention. However, until now there has been no proper scientific analysis of such cases. It is clear that we are always concerned with two completely different acts of behavior which must be defined independently. These are, first, the moment of checking or halting on something, and, second, a quite specific and fundamentally independent factor — the factor of mental activity on what was obtained as a result of the check.

Of course, there is no basis for confusion between these factors, for not distinguishing them. They are in fact completely independent acts, differing both in structure and function.

4. The Concept of Objectivization

Let us begin with the first of these factors and leave the second until the end. This first factor must be regarded as the essence of the new psychological concept which we have introduced here.

In the ceaseless course of life, during which the living being is continually changing from attempts to operate with one set to attempts to operate with another, this act of checking takes place in several cases. Instead of trying to put a particular set into operation, the subject stops, checks it, and interrupts his attempt. Instead of continuing his activity, he immobilizes it, halts it for a time. We should stress here that, instead of acting in the direction governed by his set, the subject prefers to arrest this activity, prefers to immobilize it for a short time.

But are we in fact dealing with a true cessation of the subject's activity in this case, is it in fact completely "frozen," or is this not strictly true and does he, on the contrary, continue to act as before in some way or other?

Of course, there is no such thing as a complete cessation of the working of the mind in this case. Observation shows that, on the contrary, the activity of our mind is felt particularly acutely in these cases. Instead of continuing its uniform motion forward, it halts on the spot, but not so that its activity ceases altogether, but to make an effort to re-live the event on which the check was made. This re-experience of the same event, this check, not for the purpose of experiencing nothing, of being completely inactive, but rather for making the effort to experience the same event again as happened a short time ago, this distinctive, repeated, continuing experience of the same event is the specific state of the subject in the present case. When above we described the state of re-experience of the same event, this was what we had in mind. We may conclude that in cases of active concentration on something, a subject in fact carries out this type of check on what he has just experienced. Here we experience some particular event, we experience reality as something existing independently of ourselves, as something objective. In short, we perform the act of objectivization, an act enabling us to experience something as a particular object. This is an extremely important aspect of human activity.

Not only do we experience something while acting, but we may also re-experience something or experience it for a long time.

5. The Idea of Identity or Identification

We now have a new factor which is essentially associated with this experience and which invariably follows it. Let us consider the problem of what it is that we objectivate, that we experience again as a particular object. The first idea which springs to our mind in response to this is the recognition that it is the same thing which we experience; we are conscious of the identity of the object of our experience. In this way was born the idea which subsequently developed into the axiomatic law of identity, on which as we know, the whole of our logical thought is based.

It should be remembered, however, that the idea of identity by no means coincides with what we imply by objectivization. Of course, this idea would not exist at all if there were no objectivization. However, we may also consider that objectivization would be inconceivable without the idea of identity; identity obviously assumes the presence of some form of permanent property of the object, that is, of its identity with itself. But if we observe that to objectivate something means to compare it with itself, and only that, then the idea cannot spring up in us simultaneously that this something is definitely identical with itself. For this to be possible, we must have a preliminary idea of what we should later be comparing with itself, and should thus obtain the idea of its identity with itself. It is this act of objectivization which we are stressing that gives us this idea. We must first objectivate something before we can subsequently recognize that what we have objectivated is identical with itself. Such is the psychological process of the sequence of these acts.

In short, there is a specific, psychologically independent activity which should be described as objectivization. It enables a supplementary, but essential act to take place, without which any further development would be impossible — the act of identification or the logical law of identity — an act on which the two remaining fundamental acts of our logical thought are based.

6. Speech

Turning to the next point, we must emphasize that man would find it extremely difficult to make use of his awareness of identity without the possession of speech which, by fixing this decisive achievement of thought, enabled man to reproduce it at any given moment. Speech gives us the practical possibility of manipulating identity in case of need and at will.

Without discussing these tremendous advantages of speech over any other signs which man could use to designate the fact of the identity of the objects of his thoughts, we must briefly examine the most important aspects of this problem.

When one of a number of possible experiences arises in a person's consciousness, it is abstracted in the form of speech, and the connection between speech and what it denotes is so close that there is absolutely no chance of thinking them to be independent: In the person's consciousness, they are represented as indissoluably connected. Of course, speech which expresses a particular thought may be replaced, with varying success, by different speech. But it is impossible to have thoughts and to use them repeatedly without the intervention of speech. This connection is so close and important that certain extreme tendencies exist in science (for example, behaviorism) which even go so far as to identify thought with speech. To sum up, thought, based of necessity on the principle of identity, is indissolubly connected with speech, although not of course absolutely identical with it, and Marx's formula that "language is the immediate reality of thought" expresses the objective state of affairs unusually accurately.

What do we learn from this? If, as healthy, normal persons, we have no thoughts which are independent and completely free from speech, if we have no process of thought taking place completely apart from speech, this means that fundamentally thought must have the characteristic structure of speech. Without being identical with it, it must have the same structure as speech. We have no pure thought, completely divorced from speech, and we cannot therefore state that its connection with speech is accidental and fortuitous in character. Thought is connected with speech not only in fact, but also of necessity. Not without reason did the ancient Greeks denote both by the same word.

7. Man as a Social Being

What does this mean? Speech is undoubtedly a phenomenon of social nature. It assumes the presence of a speaker and a listener, without which it would be inconceivable. Consequently, thought also must be regarded purely as a fact of a social category.

Man undoubtedly began to think and to speak when he became a member of society, for communal life and activity in society necessarily requires both. Admittedly, thought is always given to us in the form of speech, and outside this form there can be no thought as such. On the other hand, however, it is true that thought and speech are not identical phenomena, and they must be classed in two completely different categories. The fact of speech, like the fact of thought, must be preceded by its subject, the human person who tries to identify in words what he wishes to say.

The thought which is expressed is the product of the activity of a person trying to express himself in order to achieve definite goals, trying to put the thought which is present in his mind into words which will be accessible to other members of society. And so it becomes possible for a human being as an individual, to become at the same time a psychologically active participant in social life, and the mechanism of his individual mental activity thereby becomes at the same time the organ of his socially directed activity.

Hence, the need for speech, arising in man as a result of the fact of objectivization, and subsequently on the basis of identification, explains how the individual human person must be a social human person. This means that the basic psychological fact of objectivization, with the nature of which both identification and nomination are primarily associated, is essentially the product of a fundamental revolution bringing life to the development of socially determined human forms. Objectivization is essentially a social mechanism and not an individual-animal form of behavior. Objectivization is an act of behavior developing on the basis of socially determined purposes.

How is this to be understood?

The specific feature of human social life, even in the most primitive forms of its manifestation, is as follows: When man develops his activity toward the satisfaction of his needs, his concern is not limited to the strictly narrow sphere of his personal needs. He frequently steps beyond the limits of his personal needs and includes in his orbit, to some extent, attention to the interests of individuals more or less closely related to him. This distinguishes the social being from the unsocial, namely, that the circle of needs of purely personal character is supplemented by various other needs which are certainly not of this character, but are directed toward the satisfaction of the needs of a wider circle of other individuals. In the course of development of life, these social cares increase, they become the dominant form of human interests, and begin to exert a decisive influence on the whole of man's activity. The process of strengthening of this social tendency is directly related to the development of a specifically human characteristic, helping him to satisfy this tendency. I refer here to the capacity for objectivization, which has developed in man and which determines all the specific forms of his activity. As we have seen, objectivization consists essentially of the checking, the temporary arrest of the impressions acting on a person so that these impressions can be re-experienced as something objective, that is, as something existing not only for the particular person concerned, but at the same time for any other person. Naturally, by directing his activity toward phenomena and things objectivated by him, he is enabled to obtain guidance, during manipulation with these phenomena and objects, not by factors of immediate practical importance to himself, but by their objective properties, regardless of their relationship to his own purposes. This enables him to choose the direction of his activity in accordance with his own purposes and intentions. If he is concerned with the interests of another person, but not with the satisfaction of his own narrowly personal needs, the power of objectivization enables him to see the nature of his objectivated material and whether it contains anything corresponding to these interests. Objectivization gives him material which he may use, not just in accordance with his own current needs, but also in accordance with problems existing for others or which may subsequently arise to affect himself. It gives a person the power, free from the domination of personal needs necessarily acting at that particular moment, to turn his attention to the possibility of satisfying the needs of another person, or indeed of his own possible needs in the future. We could say that man became man in the true sense of the word only when, as a result of obtaining the power of objectivization and understanding the material objectivated, he became capable of escaping from the unconditional domination of the present and personal and was able to subordinate his activity to the needs and problems existing outside the sphere of the personal and present; that is, he became a man in the true sense of the word only when he acquired the ability to take trouble.

Hence, it is clear that the fundamental faculties of man — his objectivization, identification, and nomination, arising in the conditions of social life, in their turn provide the psychological condition for his further progress.

8. Repeatability as the Specific Feature of Man's External World

When studying the question of sets in animals, we found that the characteristic feature of the mental life of an animal is its constant forward movement, which continues unchecked, without any possibility of repetition. However, this happens only in animals, and the picture in man is quite different. In man, we meet a fact of cardinal importance, a fact which leaves a distinctive imprint and gives a distinctive meaning to the whole process of human life, to the whole of human activity; namely, instead of a continuous movement, in man we see checks and interruptions of this movement at various moments of his life. We see that man, having become a social being, has at the same time acquired the ability of carrying out a radical revolution in the process of his individual life, the ability to arrest its flow of ideas and to re-live it. Instead of the continuous forward course, man has acquired the power of examining reality as something concrete and repetitive. For example, he may reach the stage of beginning to contemplate the world, to experience it from an aspect of rest and immobility, as something identical to himself, something accessible to repeated perception and action. In short, because of the fundamental fact of objectivization, man is able not only to live in an objective world, but also to contemplate it as something perceived objectively. This enables him to carry out, not only practical, but also theoretical activity. This is quite impossible for an animal; the animal is unable to contemplate and cannot be concerned with theory, because psychologically speaking it is unable to objectivate.

Hence, we see that whereas the animal world appears as something continuously moving, something in a process of perpetual change, this is by no means true of man's world. The world of man must be susceptible to contemplation and it is in fact contemplated as an objective reality, as something perceived to be identical with himself and capable of being repeated any number of times. In short, it is regarded in accordance with the logical principle of identity. Because of this fact man is capable of developing a specific relationship to the outside world – he begins to perceive it. What does this mean?

9. Observation

In certain conditions, man develops a set toward a particular activity. However, as a rule he does not carry this out at once but prefers to make the set first, to objectivate the conditions of this activity, and only then starts to put these conditions into operation. When a particular set appears, man usually translates it into corresponding activity. It may happen, however, that the attempt to put it into operation is halted, either because it was a bad or unsuccessful attempt, or because it did not satisfy the need recognized in this case by the subject as, for some reason or other, more essential. It may happen, in short, that the attempt to put the particular set into operation does not satisfy the subject—for what reason is immaterial. In this case, the act of realization of the set is checked; that is, a state develops which we call objectivization, and this is immediately followed by the question: Why does the translation of the set into activity, which would be desirable in this particular case, not occur and what form must it take? It is at this stage that, as if in response to this question, the subject's intellectual activity begins, he begins to think. As a result, the subject receives the answer to his question, and he is thus shown the direction in which his activity must develop in order to give him satisfaction. We must examine this process in more detail.

In the first place, we must direct our attention to the type of mental processes which come into operation during thinking, or, in other words, we must discover what takes place in the mind on this plane of its activity, on the plane of objectivization.

To answer this question, let us take any one of a number of possible concrete, but simple, cases in our life. Let us suppose that a hunter, having seen a bird, takes aim and shoots at it. In this case, a man in the definite concrete situation of a hunter, when shooting at the bird was putting into operation the set which had developed in him in response to a given, concrete situation. Suppose he picks up the bird he has killed and sees that it is not at all what he thought it to be and quite unsuitable for satisfying his need. In any case, he must ask himself what the bird is and if, for example, he sees the same bird again, before solving the problem which interests him in this case, he must restrain himself and not shoot. In order to answer the question (What sort of bird is this?), he first begins to examine carefully the bird he has killed. This means that he will examine the individual signs of this bird: perhaps its shape as a whole, its general appearance, the color of its feathers, their shape, and various other features. The points he noticed and experienced essentially as a particular group of sensations when he saw the bird and took aim at it, he now experiences again, but this time as independent objects of his observation, as individual signs which he examines carefully and repeatedly, one after the other. We might say that in this case the subject begins to observe the bird he has killed, begins to perceive its individual signs again as properties of this bird he has killed in order that eventually he may be capable of perceiving them as signs, as properties of a particular bird. In this case, we must accept that the individual qualities which he perceives as sensory clues now become properties of the bird which he knows.

Hence, the following events take place in the hunter's consciousness: The individual qualities which he has perceived in the form of various sensations are now perceived as properties of a particular object – in this case, the bird which he knows. This result is obtained by the repeated experience of the same properties and their predication by means of speech – it results ultimately from the combined working of perception and logical (verbal) thinking, that is, from what we usually call observation.

If we now turn to our example, the power of objectivization enables the hunter, when identifying the bird he has killed, to re-experience its signs; that is, it enables him to observe the individual properties of the dead bird. This process is the first manifestation of the working of our intellect or – more precisely, it is a complex process which unifies the working of our sensation and of our verbal thinking.

10. Imagination

Following observation, a particularly important role in our mental activity is played by our ability to imagine. The whole of this process of activity, which is observed in the cases we have described, may be detected in a distinctive form in all cases of imagination. However, the specific and most characteristic form of imagination is found in the products of our memory, and we shall now discuss these.

If we turn to the animal, we have no grounds for suggesting that its memory contains imagined ideas. It is of course unquestioned that the past does not disappear completely without trace in the case of an animal – it continues to exist to some extent in its present. When, however, we speak of memory, when we say that we remember something, this means not only that we have some event from our past mental life in our present, but also that we are at the same time aware that this event in fact took place in the past and, as a rule, at a definite time in the past. The animal has no such awareness, and indeed it cannot have. The animal cannot repeat, cannot recognize identity; consequently, the animal cannot have true mnemic ideas.

It is a different matter with man. Memory is one of his most outstanding abilities, one of the fundamental psychological conditions of the birth and development of human culture.

On what is memory based?

The fundamental feature of memory is that its facts are not all experienced as original events in our mind, but as something which has already happened and is now merely being repeated. This is the fundamental sign, without which no ideas of memory would exist. Consequently, there is no doubt that the main source of the content of our mind is objectivization, which enables us to recognize identity, and also, therefore, the facts of conscious repetition, playing so important a role in the working of our memory. It is a long-established observation in science that in the process of remembering it is not simply the repetition of a particular material which plays a part, but conscious repetition. This can now be understood on the basis of our suggested explanation of the working of our memory.

Hence, memory, in the true meaning of the word, arises only on the basis of objectivization, so that it is clear that true memory is one of the specifically human faculties.

This does not mean, of course, that all the varieties of our memory must be understood to be functions of the same level of development. Analysis of the workings of our memories shows that man's mnemic ability is a structure incorporating many different levels of development and resting on the basis of objectivization. Human memory must therefore be regarded, not as a single function, qualitatively homogeneous in all its varieties, but as a faculty consisting of several different levels of development, all existing at the same time and serving, in man, several different purposes. The following varieties of workings of our minds are known: (1) passive forms — recognition, direct memory, associative memory; and (2) active forms — learning by heart and recollection. However, the way in which each of these mnemic functions works is a special problem in the psychology of memory, and we shall not discuss it further here.

11. Attention

The importance of the role ascribed in science to the specific function which we know by the name of attention is generally accepted. Analysis of the facts relating to the working of this function shows how extremely important it is in human life. However, as is usually thought, animals also must seek the help of attention. Evidently, therefore, nothing specifically human should be expected to lie at the basis of this function.

Careful analysis shows, however, that this is not the case. It may be supposed that in this connection we are dealing with a specifically human mental function, and that there are no grounds for suggesting its presence in animals. It does not seem possible to question the conscious character of the working of attention; there cannot be a case in which something could be the object of our attention, yet at the same time remain in the state of something unconscious. The essence of attention is that it is a faculty which makes conscious something which without it would remain permanently outside consciousness. There is no such thing as unconscious attention.

But how, then, can we explain the phenomena which evidently points conclusively to the presence of attention in animals? If the suggestion that conscious mental experiences exist in animals meets with insuperable difficulties, this means that the suggestion that acts of attention are possible in animals cannot be regarded as justified. For this reason, the reactions of animals which are usually considered to be reactions of attention are regarded in the science of the higher nervous activity of animals (Pavlov) as orienting responses. In response to a higher stimulus, the animal adjusts itself in the most suitable manner to deal with the situation.

If, however, it is remembered that these reactions are not purely reflex reactions, that they are definitely individual in character, and vary, not only from one individual to another, but also depending on the conditions in which they are performed, it would be easier and more correct to regard them not as reflexes in the general sense, but as reactions arising on the basis of the animal's sets. In such a case, it could be concluded that an animal is not a purely reflex being and at the same time that it is incapable of attention. The ability to perform acts of attention could then be regarded as a specifically human characteristic.

Analysis of the concept of objectivization, as we have seen above, shows that it has a very close connection with the concept of attention. It may even be considered that the link between them is so close that, from a certain point of view, no difference could be seen between these concepts. * However, a careful analysis shows that a difference is undoubtedly present between them. It is essential to distinguish between objectivization and attention, although there is no other function in man so closely connected with objectivization as attention. Nowhere, therefore, can the function of objectivization be seen so clearly as during the observations of the activities of our attention. However, it is still necessary to distinguish between them. Objectivization is merely the pause in one of our fixing states, in one of our experiences — the re-experience of something which can be made the object of our attention. Objectivization provides the material on which we can concentrate to a greater or lesser degree. If we distinguish the clarity of our experience as a specific feature of this state, then before considering the question of the degree of clarity of a given experience, we must have at our disposal a concept of the experience itself; that is, we must have a concept of some definite object, something equal and identical to the experience itself. This means that before we can discuss the degree of clarity of any of our experiences, in the first place we must have some idea concerning the experience itself, as an entity identical to itself. In other words, before we can operate our attention, we must accept the preliminary presence of the act of objectivization. Consequently, the operation of attention without the preliminary activity of objectivization is impossible.

Hence we find that processes of attention also can take place only in man as a being possessing the power of objectivization.

12. Thinking

Now let us turn to the problem of thinking. We know that for some reason or other — either because the present activity is unsuccessful or because it appears for some reason to be undesirable — a person who has halted his activity brings into operation one of his specific faculties which we call objectivization. His purpose in this case is not to put into operation his existing sets; he is not concerned with a practical problem, but rather with a problem of a theoretical order. He must determine why he is unsuccessful

*See D. Uznadze, "The Essence of Attention" (in Georgian), Psikhologiya 4 (1946).

or, perhaps, why the activity based on this particular set is apparently undesirable, and what form it should take. Hence, in the complex conditions of human life, the soil is prepared, where need be, for birth and development of activity on a theoretical plane. A subject pausing in his activity in accordance with the set in operation in these particular conditions does so in order that he may actively determine a new set corresponding to his present intentions, and take steps to put it into operation. The specific feature of this type of set is that it is the product of the subject's active efforts, his investigations in a particular direction.

What is concerned in this investigation? We have seen above that it is carried out by a specifically human faculty known as thinking. In the conditions of objectivization, the subject resorts to this type of activity, and it begins to work in order to solve the theoretical problem facing him.

Armed with all the weapons of mental activity — attention, observation, imagination of ideas — the stage is reached that at the end of a series of investigations the problem confronting the subject is finally solved. He is then faced with the question of directing his activity along the lines of the set corresponding to the meaning of the problem he has solved.

But what is this meaning in the working of our thought and, consequently, in our faculty of objectivization, if the results of this work are purely subjective and conventional in character — the same in character as the results of the sets arising directly on the basis of our needs and of the situations for their satisfaction? There would certainly be no need of objectivization or of human thought on its basis if it yielded nothing essentially new in comparison with what can be obtained by direct sets, present also in animals. Objectivization and thinking therefore arise in the conditions of man's social life, because they give him the possibility of obtaining an objectively correct solution of the problem and of adapting himself perfectly to the demands of the external environment. We might say that objectivization and the product of the social conditions of man's existence present him with the possibility of not individual, but of socially directed activity. Objectivization enables him to direct his activity on the basis of objective and correct principles: it provides man with the opportunity of recognizing the truth. Accordingly, we may conclude that man became a creative subject, transforming this world in the direction of the problems engaging him. Man became a builder of culture only after he became a thinking being and later acquired a will on the basis of objectivization.

Hence, the faculty of objectivization, presenting mankind with the opportunity for identification, nomination, and logical thought, at the same time gave him the power to carry out objectively based, correct activity, thus transforming and building this world in the direction of the interests of culture and progress.

13. The Problem of Incorrect Thinking

Does this mean, however, that thinking is always objectively based, and that cases of incorrect thinking never exist? This, of course, cannot be said. Cases of incorrect thinking are numerous, perhaps no less so than cases of correct thinking. Hence, the question arises: How can thinking of this type in general exist?

If the conditions for thinking and, above all, for objectivization are present, then it does not seem possible to explain the occurrence of incorrect thought; correctly constructed thought cannot be incorrect. Logical thought must evidently be regarded as incorrect only if it is carried out in the presence of not all the essential conditions for it, and especially in the absence of its main condition — when true and perfect objectivization does not exist.

Are such cases possible and how are they expressed? Would it be possible for the intention of investigation to be present, but if it should prove inadequate, not then give rise to complete objectivization?

The answer to these questions is clear. In the first place, there is evidence that thought processes are present in the course of man's phylogenetic development which rest on such flimsy foundations that at our levels of development they hardly appear possible. However, it also happens frequently in science that equally groundless hypotheses are encountered. Careful analysis shows that often in these cases, the course of thought, from the formal, logical point of view, is absolutely correct, although its results are in more or less clear conflict with reality. The source of the error must be not in the process of thought itself, but in the conditions in which the thought arises — the source of error must be sought in the activity of objectivization.

In what aspect of objectivization in general can the source of error be found? Clearly, objectivization as such can contain nothing which could be the source of any form of error. Objectivization itself, as we have seen above, confirms nothing and rejects nothing; it is nothing more than a fact of halting or checking a set created in a subject in the particular conditions of his activity. Consequently, in these cases there is no reason to suppose that complete and perfect objectivization is present, so that we are compelled to turn to the psychological fact which in this case appears to us as objectivization, and to examine the degree to which it can be regarded as justified by the purpose for which it appears: Can it be true that in these cases we are in fact concerned with an irrevocable fact of objectivization or, perhaps, that it is nothing more than an error, a form of self-deception of the subject?

14. "Thinking" in Mental Abnormality

To answer this question, let us examine the behavior of mentally disturbed subjects. We give below one of the many cases of the type in which we are interested.

A patient with an idea of persecution carefully examines the wall around his bed and says that he clearly sees some very suspicious lines on it. He begins to investigate the walls, conducting a series of observations on its surface, and notes the very slight bends in the lines which have been left on it accidentally. The patient concludes from his observations of these facts that there are lines on the wall around his bed which show that his persecutors havc buried an infernal machine in the wall here to blow him up when he is asleep.

It is clear from this case that the patient performs a series of attentive observations, together with thinking operations, in order to draw certain conclusions regarding the evil intentions of his enemies. Consequently, it may be concluded that in the first place he performed and act of objectivization, without which his thought processes would have been impossible.

But let us exame the peculiarity of our patient's objectivization.

If we analyze his behavior, we find that he approaches the wall around his bed with a predetermined idea — the idea that he is undoubtedly being persecuted and that he will find traces of this persecution actually on the wall — on the most suitable place from the point of view of convenience for carrying out the criminal intentions of his enemies. We see that the basis of the thought operations clearly demonstrating to our patient the presence of criminal intentions directed towards him is in this case the "objectivization" of the wall around his bed.

However, we can also see that there is no true objectivization in this case. On the contrary, the patient's consciousness is dominated by a fixed idea — the idea of his persecution, from which he cannot escape, and this idea gives a distinctive touch to the process of "objectivization" lying at the basis of our patient's intellectual operations.

It would be a great psychological error to consider that in this case in the patient's consciousness there should originally have been some type of definite idea, some precise notion of the possible methods of his persecution. This is not so; we must accept only that a set of persecution was present. And so, when he considered the wall, under the influence of this set the plot hatched against him appeared in a concrete form; he saw the lines on the wall which he took to be clues of the infernal machine hidden there.

Hence, we may conclude that the patient is completely under the power of his fixed set; he cannot escape from it even temporarily, in order to carry out true, complete objectivizations. Accordingly, the state preceding his thought operations is not one of true objectivization but one completely lacking in constant mental ideas, but by no means free from his existing fixed set. Instead of interrupting and temporarily excluding his set by checking his activity, the patient remains in its power and is thus unable to perform true objectivization.

15. Ideology

Turning now to the ordinary events of life of normal, rather than abnormal subjects, we see that the situation is often similar. The thinking of such people frequently arises on the basis of equally imperfect, defective "objectivization," such as we observed above in our diseased subject. Particularly illuminating in this direction is the question of ideology in class society. Let us examine this question in more detail.

From the subject of ideology, Engels states that "it is a process carried out by the so-called thinking man, and although it takes place with the help of consciousness, it is with the help of incorrect consciousness. The true forces exciting it and setting it in motion are unknown to it. Otherwise, this would not be an ideological process. Consequently, man creates for himself the idea of "false or illusory awakening forces" (Engels, "Letter to Mehring," in: Karl Marx, "Selected Works," Vol. 1, p. 301).

Hence, it frequently happens that man has no idea of the true sources motivating his activity — they remain hidden. However, it also happens frequently that he is forced to explain them to himself. In this case, he is aided by thought, for only thought can assist him. However, before he can start to think, the subject must check the activity of his existing set and thus make possible the act of objectivization, without which, as we have seen above, no true thought is possible.

To answer this question, we must remember that man usually follows a long path of growth and development, and clearly during this time he must produce sets of every possible type, which become fixed in him more or less securely. The sources of these sets may differ. The most important, however, are related to the action of the environment and, in particular, the class environment in which the person lives and is brought up. For instance, throughout life and, in particular during childhood, when the basis of a person's outlook is established, a series of sets is built up on the training and education he has received, and these sets accompany him, sometimes throughout life, sometimes for a shorter period. Usually, he is not aware of these sets, although this does not stop them from being active forces controlling his activity in a given direction.

Hence, in the conditions of a class society, man elaborates a series of sets directing his activity besides his consciousness. However, he may often find it necessarily to explain his actions, and this of course compels him to seek the aid of thought. Frequently, however, he is unable to carry out the act necessary for this objectivization — he cannot check or abolish these sets of which he is not aware, especially his class sets, so that he is forced to control the act of his thought under the decisive influence of these sets.

Clearly, the results of this type of thinking cannot be objectively based; they are rather the product of the subject's class set, of which as a rule he is unaware, and not the result of the operation of an objectively controlled, critically verified, unconditional thought process. Instead of determining the subject's set activity, it is itself determined by his existing set, and instead of being the result of activity based on objectivization, it is a manifestation of the pre-existing unchecked, current set. It is not the product of a thought process built up on the basis of objectivization free from unverified conditions, but the result of the activity of existing sets of which the subject is unaware.

16. Volition

Where it is a matter of complete objectivization, to put this into practice the subject turns to his volition – a new faculty arising and active in the true sense only at the human level of development. The animal has no volitional activity; it is found only in man. What has been discovered by acts of thought must be put into effect and translated into activity, and for this the corresponding powers are essential – the ability to convert the results of thought into life – in other words, the faculty of volition is necessary. Hence, we see that at the level of development of man, his active controlling force becomes his will.

But does this mean that these two extras – thought and will – are indissolubly and essentially interconnected? Observations have shown that this is not so. Cases occur in which people are not always able to do what they consider worthwhile; whereas some succeed in following the instructions of their intellect in their activity, others cannot do so. In these cases, we may speak of the force of will, and conclude that different levels of its development exist.

What is the function and what are the special features of the will? We have seen that it is the subject's power, his skill to convert into reality what his intellect considers desirable. In the animal, the situation is simple; in the presence of conditions for the satisfaction of his needs, a set appears toward suitable activity, a set which as a rule is quickly put into operation. In these cases, of course, it is a matter of the putting into operation of actually existing sets. In the conditions of working of human thought, however, there is no current set, but instead we can assume the presence of a set corresponding to the activity which is considered desirable. Consequently, the subject must activate this assumed set and put it into operation at once instead of following the set which he has checked and restrained during his act of objectivization. Thought in this case is powerless; it merely determines what must be done—but how to put into operation and make real something which exists only in the field of imagination has nothing to do with thought. This is where we see a new human faculty brought into play – the faculty of will. It is this which can convert a set to imagined activity into something real, because for a conversion of this type an effort is necessary which calls for specific conditions of upbringing and development, conditions not coinciding, moreover, with the conditions of development of the thinking faculties of man. The will makes it possible to switch over to sets regardless of what these sets promise the individual at that particular moment. The will has the power to attune a person to activity of no immediate concern for him, but of future and indirect importance.

17. Sets in Man

Let us now examine the problem of sets in man. As personal factors, as concrete attributes of the personality, at each particular moment they undoubtedly play in man just as important a role as at preceding levels of development.

Just as in other living beings, a set may appear in man, and once fixed, may continue its activity. However, this happens only when the subject is required to act in the most primitive conditions. In this case, there is no significant difference between the set in man and in other living beings.

It is a different matter in the specific conditions of human life and activity. In these conditions, we see the birth and development of sets which are possible only in the distinctive conditions of human activity. We know that in these conditions the power of objectivization is activated, and on its basis thought is born, leading man to the recognition of the need for definite types of activity. Thanks to his will, he eventually succeeds in activating a set which is found to be useful. However, during his life, man may repeatedly find himself in identical conditions, in which, in order to solve a problem, he has to seek the help of the same set. In this case, he has no need, as he did the first time, to summon the activity of objectivization, to develop acts of thought on this basis, and thus to find the required set. He can turn to the required types of set directly, without the intervention of thought, and put them into operation according to his needs.

Hence, as the field of experience widens, the range of human sets grows and extends: It includes not only sets which arise directly, but also those which the subject activated at some earlier moment of his life by means of objectivization, and put into effect by the efforts of his will.

However, this by no means exhausts the range of human sets. We must include not only sets activated for the first time on the basis of the subject's own acts of thought, but also those constructed on the basis of objectivization by unusually creative and productive personalities, and made available to mankind in general as prepared formulas, no longer requiring the direct participation of processes of objectivization. The source from which formulas of this type spring is upbringing and education, accepted as essential at each stage of development of human society. As a rule, a special period is set aside for this purpose, covering progressively longer and later sections of human life.

The acquisition of sets of this type is not confined to this period alone; it also continues later: Man's experience and knowledge continually grow and extend side by side with the corresponding skills.

Hence, the widening of the field of human sets has, in principle, no limit. It includes not only sets developing directly on the basis of current needs and situations in which they are satisfied, but also sets arising sometime in the past on the basis of personally activated or of outside objectivization, or activated by means of education — the study of the results of science and technology.

If all these facts are remembered, it is clear how widely separated are the fields of the set in man and animals. Clearly, animals have no ideas concerning objectivization — it is a characteristic limited to man. Consequently, animals can have no sets activated by objectivization. According to this principle, they have no education and, consequently, they have no opportunity of profiting by sets acquired in some way from others. The animal is restricted to the field of sets fixed during its own life, and, moreover, many of these sets are diffuse, not like those in man, which, as he undergoes development, become increasingly and more finely differentiated.

There is therefore no doubt that although sets are found in animals, and they form the basis of their activity, this does not mean that animals can be identified with man, or that they differ from man by the quantitative relationship between their powers and opportunities only. No, the specific faculty arising in man as a social individual, which we describe as the power of objectivization, produces a sharp change in the composition and character of his range of sets. Having raised man to comparatively high levels of development, this power of objectivization contributes to the subsequent increase in the complexity, the accuracy, and the degree of differentiation of his actual sets.

Consequently, the difference between man and animals in the field of sets must be regarded as extremely important; although on the other hand, it will be accepted that this difference is not a primary phenomenon, but one of arbitrary character, resulting from the properties of the specific human faculty — the properties of objectivization.

We thus see that the state of the personality, and not its individual powers and faculties, determines human behavior. In the specific conditions of his activity, particularly activity of a social character, a fundamental human faculty appears, the power of objectivization — the power to check and restrain activity, the power to halt and later to repeat it — and, on its basis, appears the power to recognize identity, followed by the power of speech. On the basis of these milestones, human thought develops, and this, making use of attention, observation, and imagination, correspondingly modified by objectivization, determines the set on the basis of which the subject, guided by his volitional effort, performs the required activity, recognized as desirable.

Thus, human psychology is built on the principle of the activity of man as a whole — on the principle of his set. The so-called mental "functions" of man — observation, imagination, and attention — like his thought and his will, are only differentiated mental properties modifying his set.

Notes From the Editor*

The monograph "Experimental Basis of the Psychology of Set" by Dmitrii Nikolaevich Uznadze (1886-1950), published in the Georgian language in 1949, was originally written by the author in Russian. This variant of the monograph is published for the first time in full in the present volume. Besides the monograph, this volume also includes D. N. Uznadze's work entitled "Basic Principles of the Theory of Set" (also written in Russian), which has not previously been published. The author's death prevented him from preparing this work finally for the press. Both texts are therefore published without editorial modifications.

Note 1

In one variant of the "Introduction," the following is also found: "How can we understand this 'faculty similar to sensation'? What had Lenin in mind when he spoke of 'a faculty similar to sensation'? It might be assumed that in this case Lenin had in mind the concept of sensation only in the sense in which it is used in modern psychology. However, the slightest observation shows that this is not so. Lenin in this case most certainly had in mind sensation not in its specific sense, not as a simple, elementary perceptual process, but as a phenomenon of general character: 'materialism regards matter as its primary fact, and regards consciousness, thought, and sensation as secondary,' says Lenin. In this case, 'sensation' is used in its broad sense — in the same sense as 'consciousness' and 'thought.' Consequently, when in this case Lenin speaks of something 'similar to sensation,' this means that he has in mind something similar also to 'consciousness' and 'thought,' although of course not identical with either of these. He has in mind a process which, while at the same time similar to various mental processes, because of this fact is not identical with anyone of these processes.

"Clearly, therefore, from Lenin's point of view, mental activity

*Of the Russian edition.

includes not only conscious processes ('consciousness, thought, sensation'), but also the stage of development which precedes them — 'a faculty similar to sensation.' "

Note 2

Most of the works listed in this bibliography as "Proceedings," "Theses," etc., were subsequently published as separate investigations.

Note 3

The following variant of the text exists:

"A simple examination of this state of affairs is sufficient to show how groundless this is. The perception of anything is itself a no less complete, independent activity than any other type of behavior. The only difference may lie in the greater or lesser complexity of the composition of the activity which we call behavior. Let us suppose that a subject, for some reason or other, develops a need to perceive something. Naturally, in this case I must distinguish, on the one hand, between need and, on the other hand, the object which must be perceived. Clearly, before perception itself arises as a fact, the subject must develop, first, a set toward perception of the particular object; otherwise he could not develop this perception. Consequently, the fact of perception cannot precede its set, but must succeed it; before a subject can carry out any definite, goal-directed act, an act of behavior in the wider meaning of the word, he must first, like the subject of this behavior, develop a certain integral state which can determine this activity. This integral state, preceding (at least logically) this type of activity and, in particular, perception, we call the set.

"Let us turn to our assumption which we stopped to interpret — the assumption that the subject, before he can use a given situation to satisfy his need — must first perceive it before producing in himself a set toward the particular activity required in this case. However, we have found that perception, in general, as an independent act of behavior, cannot precede the set; on the contrary, it requires the preliminary presence of the set. So it is also in this case: Before the subject can perceive a situation as such, in order to use it for the purpose of satisfying his need, he must already have an appropriate set; consequently, the 'perception' of the situation in this case cannot be a complete, final perception, arising as a result of an independent, complete act of 'perception.' In this case, 'perception' plays merely a subordinate role, of which the subject is not specially aware, in order to achieve some outside purpose, of dominant importance for the individual. For this reason, in this context it would be more correct to speak of the subject's noticing something rather than his perceiving it.

"Hence, when we speak, in particular, of perception we must remember that this term, strictly speaking, reflects two definite phenomena: first, the completely independent, final act of behavior, and, second, a dependent act of behavior, directly subordinated to the purposes of another, incorporating it in itself.

"It would, of course, be more correct in this second case not to mention the presence of perception at all, but to keep this term purely and simply to denote the mental phenomena implied in the first case. In the case of true perception, the problem concerned the fullest possible reflection of an object in the consciousness of the perceiving subject. In this case, perception is an independent task confronting the subject. The second type of 'perception' is another matter. In these cases, it is sufficient simply to notice the presence of the object concerned in order to go on directly to the appropriate acts of behavior. It cannot be otherwise, for in these cases the object of perception is of no independent interest to us, but merely a factor in the process of a particular activity — our purpose is not perception itself, but the particular activity for which it takes place.

"If we consider the properties of our behavior, we can easily see that the problem in this case is what form of activity must develop in order to satisfy the need arising in each individual case. Perception of an object in these cases may play only the role of a subordinate, auxiliary factor of behavior, so that no independent set is required for it. Consequently, we may assume that an active subject, besides having a particular need, from the very beginning is also endowed with a certain capacity for the preliminary noticing or 'perception,' in its distinctive meaning of the term, of the situation capable of satisfying this need."

GPSR Compliance

The European Union's (EU) General Product Safety Regulation (GPSR) is a set of rules that requires consumer products to be safe and our obligations to ensure this.

If you have any concerns about our products, you can contact us on ProductSafety@springernature.com

In case Publisher is established outside the EU, the EU authorized representative is:

Springer Nature Customer Service Center GmbH
Europaplatz 3
69115 Heidelberg, Germany

Batch number: 10844655

Printed by Printforce, the Netherlands